◆

A Practical Guide to Pharmaceutical Care

◆

Notices

The inclusion in this book of any drug in respect to which patent or trademark rights may exist shall not be deemed, and is not intended as, a grant of or authority to exercise any right or privilege protected by such patent or trademark. All such rights or trademarks are vested in the patent or trademark owner, and no other person may exercise the same without express permission, authority, or license secured from such patent or trademark owner.

The inclusion of a brand name does not mean the authors or the publisher have any particular knowledge that the brand listed has properties different from other brands of the same drug, nor should its inclusion be interpreted as an endorsement by the authors or publisher. Similarly, the fact that a particular brand has not been included does not indicate the product has been judged to be in any way unsatisfactory or unacceptable. Further, no official support or endorsement of this book by any federal or state agency or pharmaceutical company is intended or inferred.

The nature of drug information is that it is constantly evolving because of ongoing research and clinical experience and is often subject to interpretation. Readers are advised that decisions regarding drug therapy must be based on the independent judgment of the clinician, changing information about a drug (e.g., as reflected in the literature and manufacturers' most current product information), and changing medical practices.

The authors and the publisher have made every effort to ensure the accuracy and completeness of the information presented in this book. However, the authors and the publisher cannot be held responsible for the continued currency of the information, any inadvertent errors or omissions, or the application of this information.

Therefore, the authors and the publisher shall have no liability to any person or entity with regard to claims, loss, or damage caused, or alleged to be caused, directly or indirectly, by the use of information contained herein.

◆

A Practical Guide to Pharmaceutical Care

◆

*By John P. Rovers, Pharm.D., Jay D. Currie, Pharm.D.,
Harry P. Hagel, M.S., Randy P. McDonough, M.S.,
and Jenelle L. Sobotka, Pharm.D.*

*American Pharmaceutical Association
Washington, D.C.*

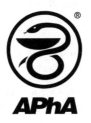

APhA

Editor: Vicki Meade, Meade Communications
Acquiring Editor: Julian I. Graubart
Layout and Graphics: Claire Purnell Graphic Design
Cover Design: Christopher K. Baker
Editorial Assistance: Cara C. Byington
Proofreading: Barbara Moss
Indexing: Mary E. Coe

©1998 by the American Pharmaceutical Association
Published by the American Pharmaceutical Association
2215 Constitution Avenue, NW, Washington, DC 20037-2985
All rights reserved.

Library of Congress Cataloging-in-Publication Data
A practical guide to pharmaceutical care / by John P. Rovers ... [et al.].

    p.   cm.
    Includes index.
    ISBN: 0-917330-90-0 (pbk.)
    1. Pharmacy—Practice. 2. Chemotherapy.   I. Rovers, John P.
    [DNLM: 1. Pharmaceutical Services—organization & administration.
    2. Delivery of Health Care—methods.   QV 737P8949 1998]
    RS100.3.P73   1998
    615' .1'068—dc21
    DNLM/DLC
    for Library of Congress   98-8812
                                                                             CIP

How to Order This Book
By phone: 800-878-0729 (802-862-0095 from outside the United States)
VISA®, MasterCard®, and American Express® cards accepted.

PRINTED AND BOUND IN CANADA BY WEBCOM LTD.

◆

Dedication

◆

This book is dedicated to our families, who have put up with our absences, both physical and mental, for far too long.

Nancy Goheen

Ann, Katheryn, and Clint Currie

Bobbie and David Hagel

Carol, Nicole, Stephanie, and Aaron McDonough

Jon, Jamie, and Drew Sobotka

Contents

Foreword

The "Iowa" pharmaceutical care vanguard has made an unparalleled contribution to the profession's migration to pharmaceutical care—in at least three ways. First, by pioneering the systematic usage of the pharmaceutical care practice model in the community setting. Second, by unselfishly sharing insights from their trailblazing "practitioner/academic" collaborative experiences with dozens of us who went on pilgrimages to their hospitable venue over the past few years. Third, by taking time to produce this compelling publication, which makes their learning available to all pharmacists.

It warms my soul to read such a straightforward account of pharmaceutical care processes and tools as is contained in this book. For practicing pharmacists yearning for seminars, workshops, and mentors, the text offers "how to" templates for implementing pharmaceutical care in any community pharmacy setting. For students trying to deal with confusing and often contradictory messages regarding pharmaceutical care, this text provides the clarification needed to understand and accept why assimilation of this new practice model is uneven. For academics, this book is a touchstone that explains authentic application of pharmaceutical care theory in the community setting.

The authors present a comprehensive, hands-on, stepwise approach to transforming the community pharmacy segment of the profession. From chapter to chapter they also lead us creatively through a detailed case study that links together the many facets of providing pharmaceutical care.

This text, and the experience it documents, convince the reader that pharmaceutical care can be successfully implemented, standardized, and remunerated in practice. Medication use can be optimized. Preventable drug-related problems can be controlled and, perhaps, eliminated altogether. And, most important, pharmacists' problem-resolution efforts can be redirected from the historical viewpoint of "What's the problem with this prescription?" to "What's the medication-related problem with this patient?"

As you read this text, be prepared to confront the obstacles hindering the progress and assimilation of pharmaceutical care. But also be ready to learn how gateways have been devised to overcome transitory opposition. The authors cover an array of cardinal and germane issues that each of us must consider—ranging from practice philosophy, attitudes, values, workflow, and changing responsibilities to marketing, planning, and compensation strategies for pharmaceutical care. The tables, charts, forms, and examples provide a rich resource for generating one's own cache of pharmaceutical care instruments.

Although converting to pharmaceutical care is a daunting experience, these Iowans have cleared the brush for the rest of us. Those with a penchant for pharmaceutical care will not be able to put this book down. Enjoy. And welcome back to patient care—we've been focusing on the pills for long enough.

Calvin H. Knowlton, Ph.D.

Past President, American Pharmaceutical Association
Co-author, *Pharmaceutical Care*[1]
Chief Executive Officer, Hospice Pharmacia, Inc., Philadelphia, PA
June 1998

1. Knowlton C, Penna D. *Pharmaceutical Care.* New York: Chapman and Hall; 1996.

◆
Preface
◆

In April of 1994, Iowa pharmacists sent a fervent message to the Iowa Pharmacists Association and Iowa's two colleges of pharmacy—The University of Iowa and Drake University. "For years," they said, "we have been dues-paying members of our association. We have been loyal alumni of our colleges, and have served as training sites for pharmacy students. Now, we need to advance our practice and our profession, and we need your help."

Consequently, the Iowa Center for Pharmaceutical Care (ICPC) was founded. The authors of this book are the original faculty and staff of the ICPC. A vital task of our center was to draw a "map"—set down in this book—that shows pharmacists how to practice pharmaceutical care.

We decided that pharmaceutical care was best illustrated by the theory of practice developed by Linda Strand and her colleagues at the University of Minnesota. They claim that pharmaceutical care focuses on patients' needs and is not necessarily a pharmacy service. The patient's need is to have drug therapy problems assessed and managed—something every clinician has done. Our job involved unbundling the tacit knowledge in this activity and describing how to address drug therapy problems systematically and consistently.

This book is the accumulated experience and knowledge that comes from having worked with several hundred pharmacists who wished to change their practices. It espouses a generalist approach to pharmaceutical care and covers patient care skills, changing the practice environment, staffing, creating the time and space to deliver pharmaceutical care, documentation, marketing, and obtaining reimbursement. Inside are answers to the difficult questions faced by any pharmacist contemplating conversion to a pharmaceutical care practice: How do I practice pharmaceutical care? Do I set up a generalist practice, or should I offer disease management programs? How can I change the practice if my employer or manager thinks it could cost more money than it will make? The book also addresses practical issues that concern any pharmacy student or teacher of pharmaceutical care. At present, there are no textbooks on pharmaceutical care practice, so reading assignments are typically drawn directly from the primary literature. Readings from a variety of sources promote diverse pharmaceutical care philosophies and ways to approach practice. Most students find these inconsistencies confusing.

Pharmacists will find the book a useful tool for teaching themselves pharmaceutical care practice or refreshing their memories on aspects of caregiving. Pharmacy entrepreneurs will benefit from the book's insights on developing the "product" in a new series of pharmacy services. Pharmacy students and teachers will value the book's practical, step-by-step approach to the care process.

GENERALIST VS. DISEASE MANAGEMENT

This book will be useful to pharmacists debating the relative merits of disease management versus generalist approaches to pharmaceutical care—which is probably the largest controversy before the profession today. Pharmacists seem to see it as an "either/or" decision, believing they can institute only one of these approaches. The authors of this book find such opinions needlessly limiting.

In our view, disease management is essentially a method to market pharmaceutical care, rather than a style of pharmaceutical care practice. We believe that the only real difference between the two approaches relates to how pharmacists define the population to whom they are providing care. For example, if a pharmacist wishes to begin an asthma management program, the process of care remains the same, except that it is limited to a single disease state.

We suggest that pharmacists begin with a generalized approach to patient care. Then, as their confidence improves—and as the marketplace warrants—they can supplement their basic competencies with a variety of disease management programs. This way, the pharmacist has the skills to look after all patients, but can also take advantage of the potentially better reimbursement climate for disease management programs.

THE EMPLOYEE PHARMACIST

Staff pharmacists who wish to practice pharmaceutical care are often in a difficult position if their employer remains skeptical. We hope that this book will help these practitioners develop a well-thought-out business proposal to share with management.

In the chain pharmacy environment, the number of decision makers increases and the difficulty of convincing them is probably greater. In that case, we would encourage staff pharmacists to develop a pharmaceutical care program and market it within their organization on a trial basis for a limited time, such as one year, to demonstrate its value.

If neither of these approaches persuades management to adopt pharmaceutical care, an option is for the staff pharmacist to focus on a narrow, well-defined population of patients and offer them at least some of the pharmaceutical care services described in this book. For example, he or she could institute a formal nonprescription drug evaluation and recommendation program for patients on anticoagulants.

Another option is to take the new skills gained from this book and use them to establish an independent, part-time pharmaceutical care practice either away from, or in cooperation with, the pharmacist's primary site of employment. Even if management is not interested in pursuing pharmaceutical care, they may be open to allowing their pharmacists to act as office- or home-based care providers if the company continues to supply products to patients.

TEACHING STUDENTS

We have long argued that, because it draws on knowledge gained from across the pharmacy curriculum, pharmaceutical care is a subject with its own curricular requirements. This book, a valuable teaching tool, represents the best attempt by experienced clinicians to describe just how they gather and use information and how they perform pharmaceutical care.

Ultimately, we hope that this book will prove useful to anyone interested in the practice of pharmacy, whatever their setting. There has been such a lot of discussion in the profession over the last few years about pharmaceutical care that sometimes the phrase seems to have lost its meaning. We hope that the consistent, clear definition of pharmaceutical care put forth in this book, and our straightforward description of how it may be practiced, will help sharpen pharmacists' understanding.

Since the 1950s our profession has been in search of a role that all pharmacists agree on and have the ability to fulfill. We believe pharmaceutical care is that role—and in this book we offer key information to help pharmacists embrace it.

◆
Acknowledgments
◆

We would like to acknowledge the ongoing support of the following individuals and organizations who have made our work possible:

The Iowa Pharmacy Foundation, Des Moines, IA

Gilbert Banker, Dean, The University of Iowa College of Pharmacy, Iowa City, IA

Stephen Hoag, Dean, Drake University College of Pharmacy & Health Sciences, Des Moines, IA

Tom Temple, Iowa Pharmacists Association, Des Moines, IA

Patti Allen, Marketing Works, Des Moines, IA

Cheryl Marsh, C. Marsh Marketing and Public Relations, Des Moines, IA

Kristen Dearden, Iowa Pharmacists Association, Des Moines, IA

Steve Firman, Iowa Pharmacists Association, Des Moines, IA

Sue Smith, Iowa Pharmacists Association, Des Moines, IA

J.R. Vallandingham, Iowa Pharmacists Association, Des Moines, IA

Michele Graves, Fifth Avenue Pharmacy and Clark's Pharmacy, Cedar Rapids, IA

In addition, we would like to thank all the leaders in pharmacy "thought" and practice, both in Iowa and across the country, from whom we learned so much.

Finally, we gratefully acknowledge the assistance of Kris Bigalk, Des Moines Area Community College, Ankeny, IA, who edited early versions of the manuscript.

◆
Contributors
◆

Jay D. Currie, Pharm.D.
Associate Professor (Clinical)
The University of Iowa College of Pharmacy
Iowa City, IA

Harry P. Hagel, M.S.
Director, Practice Management
National Health Information Network
Fort Worth, TX

Randy P. McDonough, M.S.
Assistant Professor (Clinical)
The University of Iowa College of Pharmacy
Iowa City, IA

Kevin Moores, Pharm.D.
Director, Iowa Drug Information Network, and Assistant Professor (Clinical)
The University of Iowa College of Pharmacy
Iowa City, IA

John P. Rovers, Pharm.D.
Assistant Professor of Pharmacy Practice
Drake University College of Pharmacy & Health Sciences
Des Moines, IA

Jenelle L. Sobotka, Pharm.D.
Director, Iowa Center for Pharmaceutical Care
The Iowa Pharmacists Association
Des Moines, IA

Chapter 1

◆

The Case for Pharmaceutical Care

Janice is a 43-year-old patient with diabetes. Her local pharmacy has filled her prescriptions for various oral diabetes medications for the last five years. Today she gave the pharmacist a prescription for Humulin 70/30, 35 units every morning. She is also currently being treated for glaucoma and hypothyroidism. She gets most of her other medications by mail order.

While Andy's son was picking up his father's medication at the pharmacy, he mentioned that Andy needs to be given 50 mg of Demerol by injection every night so he can sleep—a recent development in a long and complicated medical history. Andy is doing well on the current treatment and is content to continue, according to his son.

Edith called the pharmacy while the deliveryman was still at her house. She was nearly crying as she tried to explain that she couldn't afford the $45 increase in the price of her lorazepam tablets.

Pharmaceutical care is a philosophy, not forms or fixtures. At the heart it is about caring.

In each of these real-life situations, pharmacists are put in the position of making a decision. They could ignore the situation. They could acknowledge it, but do nothing to intervene. They could instruct the patient or caregiver to discuss the problem with the physician. They could attempt a quick fix with some counseling, or maybe a phone call to the physician. Or they could find out what was really going on with the patient, pinpoint unidentified problems that may exist, and work with the patient and his or her physician to make sure the appropriate care is rendered and that the patient achieves the desired effect from treatment.

ADOPTING A NEW PHILOSOPHY

Providing pharmaceutical care means adopting a philosophy of practice where pharmacists assume responsibility to choose the last of the choices on the previous page. Pharmacists take it as their duty to make sure that everything is happening in the best interest of the patient. Pharmacists must not only embrace this philosophy to provide pharmaceutical care, but must also create a work environment that allows it. A conceptual model proposed by Bernard Sorofman, shown in Figure 1, suggests the changes necessary in both the pharmacy and the pharmacist to allow organized delivery of pharmaceutical care in a pharmacy practice setting.

FIGURE 1. SYSTEMS IN PLACE VS. LACK OF SYSTEMS

		Pharmacy Site	
		Pharmaceutical care support systems in place	No support systems in place
P h a r m a c i s t	Pharmaceutical care activities	Ideal pharmaceutical care	Incomplete pharmaceutical care
	No pharmaceutical care activities	Expensive usual and customary dispensing with inadvertent pharmaceutical care	Usual and customary dispensing

Source: Sorofman BA. Iowa City, IA: The University of Iowa College of Pharmacy. Used with permission.

When pharmacists provide pharmaceutical care they use all their knowledge and skills to benefit the patient, and they provide this care to the patient over the course of time. Some basic beliefs that are important to pharmaceutical care practitioners are:

- Patients need and deserve this type of care.
- They, as pharmacists, have more to offer patients than the safe delivery of medications—they have the ability to help bring about long-term benefits to patients' health.

This level of caring for and working with the patient goes well beyond the traditional pharmacist-patient interaction. It reaches beyond the training received in pharmacy school for all but a few of the most recent pharmacy graduates. Pharmaceutical care goes hand-in-hand with a "re-professionalization" of the pharmacist and could be thought of as the pinnacle of what pharmacists have to offer patients in the health care system.

FROM PRODUCTS TO PEOPLE

In a 1986 editorial titled *Drugs Don't Have Doses—People Have Doses!*[1] Robert Cipolle defines the role of the pharmacist as a "clinical problem solver" and speaks directly to the change in practice philosophy from a product-oriented to patient-oriented profession. In 1990, Charles Hepler and Linda Strand provided the current working definition of pharmaceutical care: "The responsible provision of drug therapy for the purpose of achieving definite outcomes that improve a patient's quality of life."[2] The concepts they put forth have since been embraced by the American Pharmaceutical Association (APhA) and the American Society of Health-System Pharmacists (ASHP) as the core of their *Principles of Practice for Pharmaceutical Care* and *Statement on Pharmaceutical Care*, respectively (see Appendices, page 221). The ASHP statement defines the

---

DEFINITION OF PHARMACEUTICAL CARE

Hepler and Strand's frequently cited definition of pharmaceutical care, published in a landmark report in 1990:

> Pharmaceutical care is the responsible provision of drug therapy for the purpose of achieving definite outcomes that improve a patient's quality of life. These outcomes are (1) cure of a disease, (2) elimination or reduction of a patient's symptomatology, (3) arresting or slowing of a disease process, or (4) preventing a disease or symptomatology.

Pharmaceutical care involves the process through which a pharmacist cooperates with a patient and other professionals in designing, implementing, and monitoring a therapeutic plan that will produce specific therapeutic outcomes for the patient. This in turn involves three major functions: (1) identifying potential and actual drug-related problems, (2) resolving actual drug-related problems, and (3) preventing potential drug-related problems.

Pharmaceutical care is a necessary element of health care, and should be integrated with other elements. Pharmaceutical care is, however, provided for the direct benefit of the patient, and the pharmacist is responsible directly to the patient for the quality of that care. The fundamental relationship in pharmaceutical care is a mutually beneficial exchange in which the patient grants authority to the provider and the provider gives competence and commitment (accepts responsibility) to the patient.

The fundamental goals, processes, and relationships of pharmaceutical care exist regardless of practice setting.

Source: Hepler CD, Strand LM. Opportunities and responsibilities in pharmaceutical care. Am J Hosp Pharm. 1990;47:533-43.

mission of the pharmacist as providing pharmaceutical care, which is "...the direct, responsible provision of medication-related care for the purpose of achieving definite outcomes that improve a patient's quality of life."[3]

The APhA *Principles*[4] spell out five characteristics of pharmaceutical care:

1. A professional relationship must be established and maintained.
2. Patient-specific medical information must be collected, organized, recorded, and maintained.
3. Patient-specific medical information must be evaluated and a drug therapy plan developed mutually with the patient.
4. The pharmacist must assure that the patient has all supplies, information, and knowledge necessary to carry out the drug therapy plan.
5. The pharmacist must review, monitor, and modify the therapeutic plan as necessary and appropriate, in concert with the patient and health care team.

The concepts put forth by Hepler and Strand, APhA, and ASHP form the basis for the approach described in this book and are, we believe, prerequisites to delivering any patient care services in pharmacy. Without adopting these philosophies, a pharmacist's ability to commit the resources and effort needed to provide quality care is diminished. "Commit" is a key word, because without commitment care becomes the unorganized, sporadic delivery of isolated services to customers who are not engaged with their pharmacist.

THE THERAPEUTIC RELATIONSHIP

An integral component of pharmaceutical care is the formation of the therapeutic relationship between the pharmacist and patient. Since patients need to be actively involved in their own health care, it is essential that they develop a trusting and collaborative relationship with health care providers. In the therapeutic relationship, the pharmacist forms a covenant with the patient: a promise to do whatever possible to make sure the patient achieves positive outcomes from drug therapy. Pharmacists' contributions to this professional relationship include:

1. Holding the patient's welfare paramount,
2. Maintaining an appropriate attitude of caring for the patient's welfare,
3. Using their professional knowledge and skills on the patient's behalf.

In this cooperative relationship, the patient's responsibilities include supplying personal information, expressing preferences, and participating in the development of the care plan. The relationship is facilitated by effective communication, comprehensive data collection, and emphasis on the patient's current and future well-being. (For more information on the therapeutic relationship, see Chapter 3.)

EASIER SAID THAN DONE

Discussing definitions of pharmaceutical care and how to develop a covenantal relationship with patients is much easier than doing it. What does pharmaceutical care look like when it is implemented in practice? It *doesn't* look like consultation booths, pharmacists' offices, technicians, new computer systems, or detailed patient charts, although these are tools to facilitate pharmaceutical care. And it's not about running laboratory tests, performing pharmacokinetic calculations, answering drug information questions, or giving pharmacotherapy consults to physicians, although these are all activities that might occur in the course of providing pharmaceutical care to a patient. Pharmaceutical care is a philosophy, not forms or fixtures. At the heart it is about caring. It is about truly having concern for patients and spending the time and effort needed to help another human being.

When providing pharmaceutical care, pharmacists get to know their patients much better than ever before. They find out not only *all* the medications patients take and how they take them, but also how they feel about taking them and what they believe about their health—as well as about the role the pharmacist plays in their health. In an organized manner, the pharmacist collects and evaluates information about patients and determines what, if any, problems exist in their current therapeutic regimens. And if problems are identified, the pharmacist seeks a solution, formulates a plan to correct the problem, and puts that plan into effect to help the patient. To do this, the pharmacist may need to improve his or her skills and knowledge beyond those required for traditional pharmacy practice.

Actions the pharmacist takes might include spending time with a patient to make sure he really understands how to use his dosage form. It could be placing a call to the physician to discuss the appropriateness of a drug or dosage. Or it could mean working with the patient's care providers to develop a system to assure that she actually receives the agreed-upon medication regimen. When following up on the patient to make sure that intended outcomes are achieved, the pharmacist will seek to answer questions that, in the past, were left to others: Did the medicines dispensed actually help the patient? Is her condition resolved or as well controlled as possible? Have the therapy goals that were set been attained? Is the medication regimen causing new problems? Providing pharmaceutical care means that, at the end of the day, pharmacists measure their success by how many people they have helped, not by how many prescriptions they have filled.

A RESPONSE TO PROBLEMS IN THE SYSTEM

The reasons for the change to pharmaceutical care are many, but chief among them are deficiencies in the current drug distribution and medication use systems. A significant body of literature speaks to the negative outcomes of drug therapy on individual patients or groups of patients. Manasse[5] reviewed the causes behind the adverse consequences of medication use (his term is "drug misadventuring") and found that adverse drug reaction rates varied widely (0.66% to 50.6%). This and other reports[6,7] find that the percentage of hospitalizations due to adverse drug reactions also varies widely. Manasse concluded, perhaps conservatively, that up to 10% on average of all hospital admissions might be caused by drug misadventures. Many adverse drug reactions are not recognized as such because patients and providers may tolerate or ignore drug effects, assuming they are part of the condition under treatment or are related to some other disease.

> *Providing pharmaceutical care means that, at the end of the day, pharmacists measure their success by how many people they have helped, not by how many prescriptions they have filled.*

Many are not identified simply because no one bothered to look for them. The elderly are a group of special concern in this regard. While there is controversy regarding a link between an increased number of adverse drug reactions and increased age,[8,9] a relationship has been recognized between adverse drug reactions and an increased number of medications.[8] As the population continues to age, problems associated with adverse effects of medications will cause increasing harm to patients unless a system comes forward to address this issue.

Noncompliance with prescribed therapies is another major contributor to drug-related hospitalizations and an important cause of drug-related morbidity and mortality. A meta-analysis by Sullivan et al.[10] found noncompliance to be responsible for 5.3% of hospital admissions. A study of 315 elderly patients admitted to hospitals found that 11.4% of admissions were due to noncompliance, with 32.7% of the patients reporting a history of noncompliance in the previous year.[11] Slightly over half of this nonadherence to prescribed therapy was intentional.

Medication errors and noncompliance are also a problem in patients who have recently been discharged from the hospital. Omori et al.[12] found that 32% of patients were taking a wrong drug and 18% were taking a wrong dose one month after hospital discharge. In this study, a higher number of errors was associated with patients being on more medications at discharge or having more medication changes during hospitalization. Others have found that elderly patients on a lower than average number of medications when admitted to the hospital are at risk of being discharged with a greater increase in the number of medications than the average patient being discharged from the hospital.[13] Further need for an effective working relationship with patients was demonstrated in a study of the elderly which found that 43% of patients were unable to adhere to the prescribed regimen for one or more of their prescriptions, and that more than 70% of these intentionally did not adhere.[14]

PATIENTS' NEEDS WILL EXPAND

The growth of the nonprescription drug market from $38 billion in 1994 to $46 billion in 1995[15] and the continuing conversion of prescription drugs to nonprescription status suggests that patients' need for assistance with self-care will also continue to grow. Patients' burgeoning acceptance and use of alternative therapies, including herbal medicine, megavitamins, and homeopathy, is another indication that patients are seeking more from the health care system. A 1990 survey[16] found that visits for these therapies cost a total of $13.7 billion and exceeded the number of visits to primary care physicians. Interestingly, 75% of the cost, or over $10 billion, was paid out-of-pocket by patients for these therapies. As the most readily accessible health care providers, pharmacists can surely address this need for assistance.

Data on inappropriate prescribing also support the need for change. Willcox et al.[17] reported that 23.5% of an elderly population received one or more drugs from a list of 20 considered inappropriate for the elderly. More recently, Gonzales et al.[18] found that inappropriate use of antibiotics for conditions in which antibiotics offer little or no benefit accounted for 21% of all antibiotics prescribed to adults in 1992.

These studies provide a sense not only of opportunities for pharmacy, but also of the potential impact on health care outcomes and costs if these problems were eliminated or diminished. Some of these drug therapy problems could potentially be addressed by pharmacists in the course of providing traditional services. Rupp et al.[19] reported that 2.6% of new prescriptions presented at a community pharmacy had errors that required active pharmacist intervention. Approximately 80% of these were prescription-based errors and omissions (incomplete or vague information regarding the drug, strength, or directions). Christensen et al.[20] found that approximately 4% of prescriptions presented to an outpatient health maintenance organization contained problems, most commonly drug interactions and drug underuse. This may represent the tip of the iceberg when it comes to problems that can potentially be identified in the community pharmacy setting by pharmacists embracing a more active role.

LOWERING COSTS, IMPROVING OUTCOMES

Johnson and Bootman[21] estimated the annual cost of medication-related morbidity and mortality for the ambulatory population at $76.6 billion, noting that it matches nearly dollar for dollar the amount spent on prescription medications. According to their calculations, the cost could range from $30.1 billion to $136.8 billion, depending on the assumptions used in their model. They also estimated that because of treatment failures or new medical problems developing during therapy, more than 40% of patients would not obtain an optimal outcome of drug therapy under current conditions. In a later report, Johnson and Bootman estimated that 59.6% of the $76.6 billion could be avoided if pharmacists intervened to address drug-related problems.[22]

Although studies are limited, the literature shows that pharmacists can have an impact on both costs and patient outcomes. In one study from 20 years ago, pharmacists in six community pharmacies helped improve compliance and degree of blood pressure control in a hypertensive population study.[23] Recent studies in outpatient clinics of a university health center and a veteran's medical center, respectively, showed that pharmacists' efforts had a positive effect on blood pressure control[24] and lipids.[25] Ernst et al.,[26] who described the first year of a pharmacist-provided influenza vaccination program, noted that the pharmacist, who administered 343 doses of vaccine, contributed to an increase in immunization rates over the previous year. Currie et al.[27] found in a single pharmacy that the number of drug-related problems identified was substantially higher in a population provided pharmaceutical care than in a control group offered traditional pharmacy services. In the pharmaceutical care versus control group, the odds of detecting drug-related problems were 7.5 to 1; the odds of taking action to resolve them were 8.1 to 1. More than 57 drug-related problems per 100 patients were found in the pharmaceutical care group versus three drug-related problems per 100 patients in the control group.

Christensen et al.[28] found that giving financial incentives to pharmacists resulted in more services being documented than in a control group, and that the overall decreases in drug costs as a result of the pharmacists' actions were greater than the costs of the program. Perhaps most important, they found—as did Currie et al.—that many of the problems identified would not have been identified by automated drug use review systems. Several other studies, as well, have suggested the economic benefits[29-33] and other outcomes[22, 34-41] of pharmaceutical care.

CHANGE AND SURVIVAL

Despite the obvious need for pharmacists to expand their health care role, many are not taking steps to address the problems they are so well suited for—and the public is starting to notice. A number of articles in the lay press suggest that pharmacists do not always do all they could to protect the public's health. In Gallup polls, pharmacists are consistently rated the most trusted professionals,[42] yet recently *U.S. News and World Report* discovered that pharmacists do not always detect or intervene to prevent drug interactions.[43] Another widely publicized article pointed out that insurers sometimes exert pressure on patients and health care providers to change medication regimens in ways that may not be in the patient's best interest.[44] It is a sad fact that current reimbursement strategies and incentives often cause pharmacists to focus their attention on increasing prescription volume, maximizing efficiency, and possibly spending *less* time instead of more working with patients and their health care needs. Even Jerry Seinfeld joked in his book *Seinlanguage* that the activities he's observed pharmacists engaged in do not require a college degree.

> *...the pharmacy profession can either rally to focus on important health care needs that are not now being addressed, or it can become virtually extinct.*

Although the shift to pharmaceutical care is primarily about helping patients and addressing unmet needs, it is also about the survival of a longstanding profession. Leslie Benet conveyed the stark and uncomfortable scenario toward which pharmacy may be headed in an address to the American Association of Colleges of Pharmacy (AACP) in 1994.[45] If the trend continues of ever more prescriptions being filled by mail-order pharmacy, which technology is making faster and more efficient, only 29,200 pharmacists—one-sixth of the nation's current 170,000 total—will be needed if *all* prescriptions are eventually handled by mail order. If, however, we move instead to a pharmacist-managed medication review similar to that in a managed care facility, we will need 550,000 pharmacists, or three times the current number, to manage the country's medication needs. As Benet points out, the pharmacy profession can either rally to focus on important health care needs that are not now being addressed, or it can become virtually extinct.

This need for change is not unique to pharmacy. In his book *The Age of Paradox*, Charles Handy describes how a sigmoid curve (Figure 2) can be used to describe evolving processes.[46] As applied to pharmacy, one can see that when we controlled our professional destiny we were moving up the curve. Then outside forces created change in our environment. Competitive forces, large-volume retailers, discounters, and mail-order entered the picture. Third party payers started to reset the rules and profitability began to suffer. Our curve peaked and started to head downward. Handy contends that the secret to continued success is initiating a new curve. Pharmacists must start providing something new and unique that is both needed and desired by the health care system.

FIGURE 2. THE SIGMOID CURVE OF EVOLVING PROCESSES

This sigmoid curve can be used to describe many evolving processes, including pharmaceutical care. The height of the curve represents success and the width represents length of time. As a new process begins, uncertainties and inefficiencies take the curve in a negative direction. With time, these problems are solved and success takes the curve upward. As things continue to be done in the "same old way," while change occurs all around, the curve starts a downward shift. Point A represents the best place on the curve to start a new process. Point B represents where pharmacy is now situated.

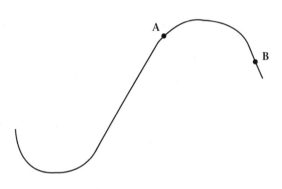

Source: Adapted from Handy C. The Age of Paradox. *Boston: Harvard Business School Press; 1994:50-67.*

Professional pharmacy groups and schools and colleges of pharmacy have recognized that pharmaceutical care is no passing trend: it's the future of pharmacy. AACP recently reaffirmed its position that the mission of pharmacy practice is to deliver pharmaceutical care.[47] AACP also recommended accelerating the pace of reforming college curricula to prepare graduates to provide pharmaceutical care.[48,49] Many colleges of pharmacy are devoting considerable resources to develop pharmaceutical care practices in community pharmacies and other health care settings.[50-53]

The window of opportunity is here now. By committing to a new form of practice and taking immediate, concrete steps, we can make pharmaceutical care a reality. For individual practitioners and students still in training, this book should provide solid tips and guidelines for launching a successful pharmaceutical care practice.

REFERENCES

1. Cipolle RJ. Drugs Don't Have Doses–People Have Doses! A Clinical Educator's Philosophy. *Drug Intell Clin Pharm.* 1986;20:881-2.

2. Hepler CD, Strand LM. Opportunities and responsibilities in pharmaceutical care. *Am J Hosp Pharm.* 1990;47:533-43.

3. American Society of Hospital Pharmacists. ASHP statement on pharmaceutical care. *Am J Hosp Pharm.* 1993;50:1720-3.

4. *Principles of Practice for Pharmaceutical Care.* Washington, DC: American Pharmaceutical Association; 1995.

5. Manasse HR. Medication use in an imperfect world: drug misadventuring as an issue of public policy, Part 1. *Am J Hosp Pharm.* 1989;46:929-44.

6. McKenney JM, Harrison WL. Drug-related hospital admissions. *Am J Hosp Pharm.* 1976;33:792-5.

7. Caranasos GJ, Steward RB, Cluff LE. Drug-induced illness leading to hospitalization. *JAMA.* 1974;228:713-7.

8. Gurwitz JH, Avorn J. The ambiguous relation between aging and adverse drug reactions. *Ann Intern Med.* 1991;114:956-66.

9. Nolan L, O'Malley K. Prescribing for the elderly: Part I, Sensitivity of the elderly to adverse drug reactions. *J Am Geriatr Soc.* 1988;36:142-9.

10. Sullivan SD, Kreling DH, Hazlet TK. Noncompliance with medication regimens and subsequent hospitalization: a literature analysis and cost of hospitalization estimate. *J Res Pharm Econ.* 1990;2:19-33.

11. Col N, Fanale JF, Kronholm P. The role of medication noncompliance and adverse drug reactions in hospitalizations of the elderly. *Arch Intern Med.* 1990;150:841-5.

12. Omori DM, Potyk RP, Kroenke K. The adverse effects of hospitalization on drug regimens. *Arch Intern Med.* 1991;151:1562-4.

13. Beers MH, Dang J, Hasegawa J, Tamai IY. Influence of hospitalization on drug therapy in the elderly. *J Am Geriatr Soc.* 1989;37:679-83.

14. Cooper JK, Love DW, Raffoul PR. Intentional prescription nonadherence (noncompliance) by the elderly. *J Am Geriatr Soc.* 1982;30:329-33.

15. Anon. OTC drug market shows strong growth. *NARD Newsletter.* 1997;119(1):1.

16. Eisenberg DM, Kessler RC, Foster C, et al. Unconventional medicine in the United States: prevalence, costs and patterns of use. *N Engl J Med.* 1993;328:246-52.

17. Willcox SM, Himmelstein DU, Woolhandler S. Inappropriate drug prescribing for the community-dwelling elderly. *JAMA.* 1994;272:292-6.

18. Gonzales R, Steiner JF, Sande MA. Antibiotic prescribing for adults with colds, upper respiratory tract infections, and bronchitis by ambulatory care physicians. *JAMA*. 1997;278:901-4.

19. Rupp MT, Schondelmeyer SW, Wilson GT, et al. Documenting prescribing errors and pharmacist interventions in community pharmacy practice. *Am Pharm*. 1988;NS28(9):30-7.

20. Christensen DB, Campbell WH, Madsen S, et al. Documenting outpatient problem intervention activities of pharmacists in an HMO. *Med Care*. 1981;19:104-16.

21. Johnson JA, Bootman JL. Drug-related morbidity and mortality: a cost-of-illness model. *Arch Intern Med*. 1995;155:1949-56.

22. Johnson JA, Bootman JL. Drug-related morbidity and mortality and the economic impact of pharmaceutical care. *Am J Health-Syst Pharm*. 1997;54:554-8.

23. McKenney JM, Brown ED, Necsary R, Reavis HL. Effect of pharmacist drug monitoring and patient education on hypertensive patients. *Contemp Pharm Prac*. 1978;1(2):50-6.

24. Erickson SR, Slaughter R, Halapy H. Pharmacists' ability to influence outcomes of hypertension therapy. *Pharmacotherapy*. 1997;17:140-7.

25. Konzem SL, Gray DR, Kashyap ML. Effect of pharmaceutical care on optimum colestipol treatment of elderly hypercholesterolemic veterans. *Pharmacotherapy*. 1997;17:576-83.

26. Ernst ME, Chalstrom CV, Currie JD, Sorofman B. Implementation of a community pharmacy-based influenza vaccination program. *J Am Pharm Assoc*. 1997;NS37:570-80.

27. Currie, JD, Chrischilles EA, Kuehl AK, Buser RA. Effect of a training program on community pharmacists' detection of and intervention in drug-related problems. *J Am Pharm Assoc*. 1997;NS37:182-91.

28. Christensen DB, Holmes GH, Andrews A, et al. Payment of pharmacists for cognitive services: results of the Washington State C.A.R.E. demonstration project. Medical Assistance Administration Department of Social and Health Services State of Washington, Department of Pharmacy, School of Pharmacy, University of Washington. December 1996.

29. Hatoum HT, Catizone C, Hutchinson RA, Purohit A. An eleven-year review of the pharmacy literature: documentation of the value and acceptance of clinical pharmacy. *Drug Intell Clin Pharm*. 1986;20:33-41.

30. Willett MS, Bertch KE, Rich DS, Ereshefsky L. Prospectus on the economic value of clinical pharmacy services. *Pharmacotherapy*. 1989;9:45-56.

31. Schumock GT, Meek PD, Ploetz PA, et al. Economic evaluation of clinical pharmacy services 1988-1995. *Pharmacotherapy*. 1996;16:1188-208.

32. Dobie RL, Rascati KL. Documenting the value of pharmacist interventions. *Am Pharm.* 1994;NS34:50-4.

33. Rupp MT. Value of community pharmacists' interventions to correct prescribing errors. *Ann Pharmacother.* 1992;26:1580-4.

34. Martin S. Pharmaceutical care made easy. *Am Pharm.* 1994;NS34(3):61-4.

35. Meade V. Pharmaceutical care in a changing health care system. *Am Pharm.* 1994;NS34(8):43-6.

36. Meade V. Adapting to providing pharmaceutical care. *Am Pharm.* 1994; NS34(10):37-42.

37. Meade V. Pharmacist in Richmond launches pharmaceutical care program. *Am Pharm.* 1994;NS34(11):43-5.

38. Meade V. Helping pharmacists provide disease-based pharmaceutical care. *Am Pharm.* 1995;NS35(3):45-8.

39. Bloom MZ. Simple changes reap big rewards. *Am Pharm.* 1995;NS35(8):18-9.

40. Tomechko MA, Strand LM, Morley PC, Cipolle RJ. Q and A from the pharmaceutical care project in Minnesota. *Am Pharm.* 1995;NS35(4):30-9.

41. Grainger-Rousseau TJ, Miralles MA, Hepler CD, et al. Therapeutic outcomes monitoring: Application of pharmaceutical care guidelines to community pharmacy. *J Am Pharm Assoc.* 1997;NS37(6):647-61.

42. Anon. Community pharmacists top Gallup poll. *NARD Newsletter.* 1997; 119(2):2.

43. Headden S, Lenzy T, Kostyu P, et al. Danger at the Drugstore. *U.S. News & World Report.* August 25, 1996:46-53.

44. Headden S. The big pill push. *U.S. News & World Report.* September 1, 1997:67-75.

45. Benet LZ. Pharmacy education in an era of health care reform. *Am J Pharm Educ.* 1994;58:399-401.

46. Handy C. *The Age of Paradox.* Boston: Harvard Business School Press; 1994:50-67.

47. Commission to Implement Change in Pharmaceutical Education. Maintaining our commitment to change. American Association of Colleges of Pharmacy. Alexandria, VA. (January 1997).

48. Commission to Implement Change in Pharmaceutical Education. Background Paper I: What is the Mission of Pharmaceutical Education? *Am J Pharm Educ.* 1993;57:374-6.

49. Commission to Implement Change in Pharmaceutical Education. Background Paper II: Entry Level, Curricular Outcomes, Curricular Content and Educational Process. *Am J Pharm Educ.* 1993;57:377-85.

50. Currie JD, McDonough RP, Hagel HP, et al. College of Pharmacy faculty time spent developing pharmaceutical care practice sites [Abstract]. *Pharmacotherapy*. 1996;16:141.

51. Rovers J, Hagel H, McDonough R, Currie J. Impact on college faculty of implementing pharmaceutical care in community pharmacies [Abstract]. *Pharmacotherapy*. 1996;16:140.

52. Hagel H. Expanding clinical practice to community pharmacy settings [Abstract]. *Pharmacotherapy*. 1996;16:140.

53. Kennedy DT, Ruffin DM, Goode JR, Small RE. The role of academia in community-based pharmaceutical care. *Pharmacotherapy*. 1997;17(6):1352-6.

Chapter 2

◆

Identifying Drug Therapy Problems

The goal of the pharmaceutical care pharmacist is to prevent drug therapy problems before they occur and to resolve problems that already exist. As explained in APhA's *Principles of Practice for Pharmaceutical Care*, the pharmacist works in concert with the patient and the patient's other health care providers to promote health, prevent disease, and assure that drug therapy regimens are safe and effective.[1] Pharmacists who practice in a pharmaceutical care setting share their expertise in the area of drug therapy problems to promote the health and well-being of patients.

This chapter and the three that follow it cover how this is done and give concrete information to help pharmacists develop practical skills for providing pharmaceutical care.

THE PHARMACEUTICAL CARE CYCLE

The practice of pharmaceutical care involves an ongoing series of steps, as illustrated in the diagram of the Care Cycle. The entry point to the cycle is identifying a drug therapy problem.

In the Care Cycle, the pharmacist initially asks himself why he should act—does the patient have a drug therapy problem? If the answer is yes, then the pharmacist should be roused into action. His next step is to determine what he would like to do about it, which involves setting a therapeutic goal for the patient. After that, he must decide how best to achieve the goal. At this point, the pharmacist develops and implements a care plan. After the plan is in place, the final step is to perform adequate patient follow-up and monitoring to determine if the therapeutic goal has been achieved.

If the goal has been accomplished, the cycle stops until the next time the pharmacist has a reason to evaluate the patient. If the goal has not been achieved, or if the patient subsequently develops a new drug therapy problem, the Care Cycle begins again. Each time the pharmacist detects a drug therapy problem, it is a cue for him to act.

FIGURE 1. THE CARE CYCLE

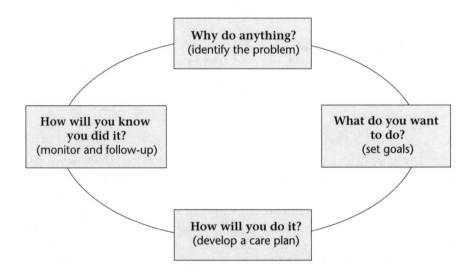

Source: Rovers J. Des Moines, IA: Drake University College of Pharmacy. Used with permission.

DRUG THERAPY PROBLEMS, NOT MEDICAL PROBLEMS

It is important to understand the difference between medical problems and drug therapy problems. A medical problem is a disease state: that is, a problem related to altered physiology resulting in clinical evidence of damage. A drug therapy problem, however, is a patient problem that is either caused by or may be treated with a drug. Drug therapy problems typically develop out of medical problems. Hypertension is a disease, and therefore is a medical problem. If a patient requires drug therapy for her hypertension and is not receiving it, she has a drug therapy problem. The *hypertension* is not the drug therapy problem, but *the need* for drug therapy is.

In practice, such distinctions are essential. The diagnosis of a medical problem is the responsibility of the physician, whereas the scope of a pharmacist's practice must be limited only to drug therapy problems. After a pharmacist has provided pharmaceutical care to a few patients, he can readily distinguish between the two types of problems. Until then, however, practitioners must use extreme caution to ensure that they are not inadvertently trying to diagnose medical conditions—which is clearly the role of a physician. They must also not allow themselves to be drawn into discussions of diagnostic medicine when patients ask for the pharmacist's opinion about their disease states.

DISCOVERING DRUG THERAPY PROBLEMS

When pharmacists critically evaluate their current practice, it is readily apparent that they already find and solve drug therapy problems. Each day, pharmacists discover drug interactions and therapeutic duplications, speak to physicians, educate patients, and do what is necessary to solve the problems they uncover. Are such pharmacists practicing pharmaceutical care? The answer lies, in part, in how the average pharmacist currently uncovers drug therapy problems and how the pharmaceutical care practitioner completes the process after a drug therapy problem is identified.

> *Medical problems* are disease states; that is, problems related to altered physiology that result in clinical evidence of damage.
>
> *Drug therapy problems* are problems patients are undergoing that are either caused by a drug or may be treated with a drug.

Typically there are only a limited number of ways in which pharmacists become aware that a patient has a problem related to a drug. Usually it is when a pharmacist looks down at the prescription she is filling and thinks, "That can't be right!" This is especially true for problems related to dose, dosage interval, or duration of therapy. Alternatively, many drug therapy problems are identified when the drug utilization review module of the pharmacist's dispensing software or the third party payer's claims computer indicates a possible drug interaction, therapeutic duplication, or compliance problem.

All problems identified by these methods have two features in common: *they represent a problem with a prescription, not a patient with a problem.* Furthermore, none represents problems that the pharmacist necessarily intended to find; rather they are things she came upon in the routine course of filling a prescription. At the risk of sounding uncharitable, right now pharmacists do not find problems so much as problems find pharmacists. The discovery of these problems is not always purposeful or organized, but often accidental.

An organized approach is critical to success. A study by Currie et al. shows that when problems were identified by the usual methods, pharmacists found an average of three drug therapy problems per 100 patients.[2] However, when trained pharmacists set out with the *intention* of looking for drug therapy problems, they found an average of 57.6 problems per 100 patients. Overall, pharmacists who used an organized approach were 7.5 times more likely to find a drug therapy problem than pharmacists identifying problems using the more usual methods.

More Than Profile Review Needed

Not all drug therapy problems can be identified from the prescription, a profile review, and screening software. Pharmaceutical care practitioners make a point of gathering additional information to ensure that the intended outcome of therapy is achieved and that no drug therapy problems occur.

In a pharmaceutical care practice, pharmacists set out with the *intention* of looking for problems that they would not or could not otherwise identify. Consider the following examples. A pharmacist fills a prescription for amoxicillin 250 mg capsules to be taken three times a day for 10 days. While performing a routine review of the patient's medication profile, the pharmacist notices that the patient is also taking an oral contraceptive. The pharmacist correctly identifies a potential drug interaction and counsels the patient on the need for an alternative method of birth control for the rest of the month. In a slightly different scenario, the same pharmacist fills the same prescription and performs the same profile review, but does not find a potential drug interaction or anything to suggest the patient uses oral contraceptives. The patient receives standard counseling about her medication. Later she becomes unintentionally pregnant because the amoxicillin interfered with the effectiveness of birth control pills she received as physician samples—which the pharmacist did not know she was taking. Without more patient-specific knowledge, the pharmacist could not identify the potential drug interaction.

The pharmaceutical care provider knows that not all problems can be identified from the prescription, a profile review, and screening software. Such practitioners make a point of gathering additional information to ensure that the intended outcome of therapy is achieved and that no drug therapy problems occur.

So, in answer to the question about whether pharmacists who discover problems provide pharmaceutical care, it would appear that most of these practitioners are *partial* providers of pharmaceutical care. But without a more formal understanding of what drug therapy problems are and how to find them in a consistent, logical, and organized fashion, pharmacists cannot identify all such problems and provide the level of care their patients require.

BEYOND COUNSELING

The APhA *Principles of Practice for Pharmaceutical Care* describes five steps to the pharmaceutical care process (see box).[1] As a pharmacist carries out the activities required to perform each of these steps, he is practicing pharmaceutical care.

Drug therapy problems may be identified during steps 2 and 3, since this is where the pharmacist gathers patient-specific data and critically examines it to determine if problems exist. Implicit in these five steps is the reality that providing pharmaceutical care requires an entire shift of focus for the pharmacy practice; instead of focusing on product alone, the pharmacist must accept a new level of responsibility. In the past, in traditional dispensing practices, pharmacists were simply responsible for dispensing prescriptions accurately, as prescribed. When Congress passed a law in 1990 requiring that pharmacists provide medication counseling to Medicaid patients about their prescriptions (known as "OBRA '90"), and states subsequently amended their pharmacy practice acts to require such counseling for *all* patients obtaining prescription medications, pharmacists assumed responsibility for ensuring that patients understand key aspects of the use of medications. In providing pharmaceutical care, the pharmacist goes far beyond this to assume responsibility for all the patient's drug-related needs. These needs are summarized in the box to the right.

FIVE STEPS IN THE PHARMACEUTICAL CARE PROCESS

1. A professional relationship with the patient must be established.
2. Patient-specific medical information must be collected, organized, recorded, and maintained.
3. Patient-specific medical information must be evaluated and a drug therapy plan developed mutually with the patient.
4. The pharmacist must ensure that the patient has all supplies, information, and knowledge necessary to carry out the drug therapy plan.
5. The pharmacist must review, monitor, and modify the therapeutic plan as necessary and appropriate, in concert with the patient and health care team.

FIVE KEY DRUG-RELATED NEEDS OF PATIENTS

Pharmacists who provide pharmaceutical care must ensure that the following needs are met:

1. Patients have an appropriate indication for every drug they are taking.
2. Patients' drug therapy is effective.
3. Patients' drug therapy is safe.
4. Patients can comply with drug therapy and other aspects of their care plans.
5. Patients have all drug therapies necessary to resolve any untreated indications.

As the list suggests, the pharmacist must be certain that every medication being taken is for a legitimate purpose and that the drug is achieving the desired therapeutic goals—without undue risk of adverse effects or drug interactions. The pharmacist must also verify that the patient is able to carry out the drug regimen as instructed and that the patient has no additional untreated conditions that would benefit from adding drug therapy. The five drug-related needs are associated with seven types of drug therapy problems (see Table 1). Only after each of these five needs has been evaluated and the pharmacist feels confident that each is being met in the optimal fashion can she conclude that the patient does not have a drug therapy problem.

TABLE 1. PROBLEMS RESULTING FROM UNMET DRUG-RELATED NEEDS

Drug-Related Need	Drug Therapy Problem
Appropriate indication	1. Unnecessary drug therapy
Effectiveness	2. Wrong drug
	3. Dosage too low
Safety	4. Adverse drug reaction
	5. Dosage too high
Compliance	6. Inappropriate compliance
Untreated indication	7. Needs additional drug therapy

Source: Tomechko MA, Strand LM, Morley PC, Cipolle RJ. Q and A from the pharmaceutical care project in Minnesota. Am Pharm. 1995;NS35(4):30-9.

CAUSES OF DRUG THERAPY PROBLEMS

As pharmacists gather history, evaluate data, and identify drug therapy problems, they must also determine the cause of each problem. The cause is important because it suggests potential therapeutic plans that may be implemented to solve the problem. An extra few minutes determining the cause can prevent the pharmacist from developing a plan that does not ultimately assist the patient. Each of the drug therapy problems in Table 1 has a limited number of causes, as shown in Table 2.

Both tables provide powerful evidence that present methods of problem identification are insufficient. Although the methods commonly used in pharmacies today may allow pharmacists to identify occasional problems with prescriptions related to compliance, allergies, drug interactions, etc., not all problems and causes can be identified without further data. For example, it would be impossible for a pharmacist to determine if additional drug therapy is needed unless he is aware of the patient's current medical conditions.

TABLE 2. CAUSES OF DRUG THERAPY PROBLEMS

Drug Therapy Problem	Cause
Unnecessary drug therapy	No medical indication Addiction/recreational drug use Nondrug therapy more appropriate Duplicate therapy Treating avoidable adverse reaction
Wrong drug	Dosage form inappropriate Contraindication present Condition refractory to drug Drug not indicated for condition More effective drug available
Dosage too low	Wrong dosage Frequency inappropriate Duration inappropriate Incorrect storage Incorrect administration Drug interaction
Adverse drug reaction	Unsafe drug for patient Allergic reaction Incorrect administration Drug interaction Dosage increased or decreased too quickly Undesirable effect
Dosage too high	Wrong dose Frequency inappropriate Duration inappropriate Drug interaction
Inappropriate compliance	Drug product not available Cannot afford drug product Cannot swallow or otherwise administer drug Does not understand instructions Patient prefers not to take drug
Needs additional drug therapy	Untreated condition Synergistic therapy Prophylactic therapy

Source: Tomechko MA, Strand LM, Morley PC, Cipolle RJ. Q and A from the pharmaceutical care project in Minnesota. Am Pharm. *1995;NS35(4):30-9.*

A pharmaceutical care approach to practice is required to be able to identify *a patient with a problem*, rather than *a problem with a prescription*. Without this approach, only a small proportion of drug therapy problems will be discovered and acted upon. And even if a problem is identified, without adequate data it is difficult to determine why the problem occurred. In such a case, there is little the pharmacist can do but provide further patient counseling and emphasize the need for compliance. A pharmaceutical care practitioner, however, could determine if the patient is noncompliant because he has had an adverse effect, cannot afford the drug, or simply does not believe that the drug works. Once the cause is known, the appropriate educational intervention becomes more apparent.

'ACTUAL' AND 'POTENTIAL' DRUG THERAPY PROBLEMS

Drug therapy problems may be actual or potential. The distinction between the two is important, but is not always immediately apparent in practice. An *actual* problem is one that has already occurred, and thus the pharmacist must try to fix it. A *potential* problem is one that is likely to occur—something the patient is at risk of developing—if the pharmacist makes no intervention. When an actual drug problem exists, the pharmacist should take immediate action. If there is a potential drug problem, the pharmacist should take the necessary steps to prevent it.

Is the following problem actual or potential? A pharmacist is counseling a patient about a new amoxicillin prescription and learns that he has a history of immediate hypersensitivity reactions to penicillin. As shown in Table 2, this problem would be identified as an adverse drug reaction caused by an allergic reaction. The problem is *potential*, since the patient did not actually suffer an allergic reaction to the new prescription. Now suppose the patient actually took the amoxicillin. Again, unless the patient develops signs and symptoms of an allergic reaction, the problem remains potential.

The pharmacist may also identify a problem as potential if he suspects that a problem exists but has not yet obtained sufficient data to identify it definitively as a problem. Suppose, for example, that after screening a patient's profile a pharmacist believes her to be noncompliant with her high blood pressure medication. Until the pharmacist can definitely confirm that she is not taking the medication as directed, this problem remains a potential one.

COMMUNICATION TIP: PAY ATTENTION TO WORD CHOICE

Special attention must be paid to the words used to define certain problems and causes. Phrases such as "wrong drug" or "duration inappropriate" may be accurate in describing the patient's problem, but they carry a negative connotation when the pharmacist uses them while discussing the problem with others, especially physicians. When communicating with the physician about a drug therapy problem, it is critical to remember that pharmaceutical care is new for the rest of the health care system, and as such, is a potential threat. Human beings work in that system, and they may not appreciate a pharmacist's opinion that the "wrong drug" was prescribed. Sometimes, phrasing a problem as a question may be more socially acceptable. For example:

• A pharmacist fills a prescription for hydrochlorothiazide 100 mg tablets to be taken once daily. Since the dose appears to be high, she confirms with the patient that the drug is for mild hypertension that has just been diagnosed. The patient has never tried other drugs for his blood pressure. The pharmacist contacts the physician's office and informs the nurse that the dosage of hydrochlorothiazide is "too high." A few minutes later, the nurse calls back, sounding annoyed, and simply confirms that the physician wants a dosage of 100 mg.

Now imagine the same clinical scenario, with a few changes.

• The pharmacist phones the physician's office and tells the nurse that she does not often see 100 mg hydrochlorothiazide dosages and would like to clarify how the dosage was selected so that she may better understand how the physician intends to treat this patient. She also indicates that this knowledge will assist her in helping the patient achieve the outcome the physician intends. Depending on the answer received, this more low-key approach allows the pharmacist to recommend a new dosage that "may have less risk of side effects," or "may be just as effective and may be safer."

In both cases, the same problem is identified. In the second case, however, the problem was communicated in a way that is less likely to be interpreted as negative. A physician who is not placed on the defensive because the drug therapy problem is poorly worded is more likely to be receptive to a pharmacist's suggestions.

As the pharmaceutical care marketplace develops, the value of organizing drug therapy problems by patient need, resultant problem, and attendant cause is likely to play a role in how pharmacists document care. Although physicians may occasionally take umbrage at how drug therapy problems are worded, payers and quality assurance bodies have a substantial interest in the precise nature and causes of the problems seen in practice and are less emotionally invested in judgments of "right" and "wrong." Such data allow them to develop appropriate risk management tools to minimize further risk of drug therapy problems. The implication for pharmacists is essentially this: document the problem fully, but be careful with the wording when presenting it to other health care providers.

The concept of actual and potential problems can be a sticky issue in the pharmacist-physician relationship. In the typical pharmacy practice, most interventions that pharmacists try to make with prescribers are related to potential problems. Oftentimes, physicians do not take potential problems as seriously as pharmacists do. One common example is drug-drug interactions. Unless the patient is actually suffering from toxicity or lack of clinical effect because of a drug-drug interaction, this is a potential drug therapy problem. All too often, the pharmacist informs the physician of such a potential problem only to find that the physician continues with the original therapy. To most physicians, unless the interaction is potentially lethal, such as an interaction involving warfarin, potential problems are exactly that—*potential*. The consequences of a potential problem must often be very severe before the physician is motivated to act.

The outcome is usually different in pharmacist-physician interactions involving actual drug therapy problems. For example, if a pharmacist discovers that a patient is noncompliant with his expensive cholesterol-lowering agent because he cannot afford it, the physician is typically more motivated to switch to an agent that the patient will be able to comply with. With a problem like this, the physician knows that unless it is fixed, the intended outcome of therapy will not be achieved.

All this having been said, pharmacists should not conclude that potential problems do not require action. Rather, before deciding to contact the physician they should consider how severe the consequences of the potential problem could be. The consequences of prescribing penicillin to a patient who has had a previous allergic reaction to penicillin are far different from those of giving ibuprofen to a patient with a history of mild gastric upset from ibuprofen. In both cases the pharmacist should still act on the problem, but the latter is less likely to require the physician's intervention. Most pharmacists already try to eliminate unnecessary phone calls to physicians by setting the threshold of their drug interaction screening software high enough so only clinically relevant interactions are likely to be flagged. As pharmacists develop into full-fledged pharmaceutical care practitioners, they will treat a wider variety of drug therapy problems in a similar manner.

Although finding and resolving drug-related problems requires a new thought process, it isn't far removed from the thought processes of all pharmacists. Pharmacists are already trained to examine prescriptions and identify potential problems; pharmaceutical care takes this process one step further, to the patient. The most challenging aspects of providing pharmaceutical care are learning to focus on the patient, ask the right questions, and develop good investigative and research skills.

CASE STUDY

The case at the right will be considered over the next few chapters. After reading it, take time to consider the questions at the end. These questions force the pharmacist to think about ways to determine if the patient's needs are being met and the kind of information that must be collected to identify drug therapy problems that may exist. By answering these questions, the pharmacist begins the first step in providing pharmaceutical care.

REFERENCES

1. *Principles of Practice for Pharmaceutical Care.* Washington, DC: American Pharmaceutical Association; 1995.

2. Currie JD, Chrischilles EA, Kuehl AK, Buser RA. Effect of a training program on community pharmacists' detection of and intervention in drug-related problems. *J Am Pharm Assoc.* 1997;NS37:182-91.

CASE STUDY

Mary Blythe is a white female in her mid-30s who is a new patient in your pharmacy. You have never filled a prescription for her before. Today, Mary presents you with a new prescription for Serzone (nefazodone) 150 mg tablets, Sig: 1 tablet twice daily, refill X 3, signed by Dr. R. Dennis, a local family physician. Mary also wishes to purchase a bottle of Afrin (oxymetazoline) Nasal Spray. As you gather the usual demographic and insurance data, you learn that Mary has prescription insurance through her husband's employer and has a $10 copay on each prescription. She is employed as a real-estate agent in a local office and she has a 14-year-old son. There is nothing in Mary's mood, behavior, dress, or appearance to suggest that anything is abnormal. She appears to be about 5' 5" tall, and her weight appears normal for her height.

1. *How should the pharmacist begin to develop a therapeutic relationship with the patient so that he is able to start collecting the data needed to identify any drug therapy problems?*

2. *What data need to be collected to determine if:*
   a) *there is an appropriate indication for each drug;*
   b) *the drug therapy is effective;*
   c) *the drug therapy is safe;*
   d) *the patient is able to comply with the drug therapy;*
   e) *there are any untreated conditions that should be treated with drug therapy?*

Chapter 3
◆
Patient Data Collection

In this chapter, the major topics covered are history taking and data gathering, including types of data, how data may be collected using patient interviews and other tools, and specific data that are needed to provide pharmaceutical care. Subsequent chapters will be devoted to how to assess the data collected and how to develop and implement care plans.

The pharmacist's initial interview with the patient establishes the professional relationship and initiates the patient's pharmacy record. The purpose of the interview is to help build a comprehensive database and develop a good working knowledge of the patient's total health picture. Sometimes it may be necessary to gather information over a series of interviews, rather than one long interview. Interviews that take place after the initial interview should focus on updating existing information and gathering new information, as needed.

As this chapter suggests, collecting accurate, comprehensive patient information involves much more than a quick consultation in which a patient fills out a form. For data to be collected successfully, there must be a strong, professional relationship between pharmacist and patient. This relationship is characterized by caring, trust, open communication, cooperation, and mutual decision-making. The insightful pharmacist who focuses on the patient, asks good, open-ended questions, and listens attentively will find that professional relationships with patients can readily be achieved.

SUBJECTIVE VS. OBJECTIVE

Both objective and subjective data are typically collected as a basis for pharmaceutical care. Subjective information cannot be measured directly and may not always be accurate or reproducible. Subjective data are often supplied directly by the patient, such as the patient's medical history, chief complaint, history of the present illness, general health and activity status, and social history. Pharmacists are limited in their ability to confirm the accuracy of data the patient provides. Objective data can be measured, are observable, and are not influenced by emotion or prejudice. Much objective information is numerical. Examples are vital signs and laboratory measures of substances such as blood lipids.

Whether medication history is subjective or objective is a topic of debate. Many pharmacists consider it to be subjective data since it is part of the patient's history and is typically gathered directly from the patient. Others feel that, as the only health care practitioners trained to gather a medication history, in their hands this information is consistently measurable. The same argument may be made for history related to compliance. Many trained practitioners assume compliance data are objective because they assess such information every day.

Although laboratory data are typically considered to be objective, it depends on the source of the information. If a patient tells the pharmacist that his doctor said his cholesterol is 255 mg/dl, it is not objective information unless the pharmacist can confirm it. On the other hand, if the same patient shows the pharmacist a lab results slip with the same information on it, the source of the information is objective. Strictly speaking, unless the pharmacist receives laboratory values from the physician's office or lab, or can verify results against a slip the patient supplies, patient-supplied data are subjective. Increasingly, however, pharmacists are collecting their own objective data. Tests for peak expiratory flow rates, blood pressures, serum glucose levels, and serum lipid profiles are now commonly done in the pharmacy and provide the practitioner with truly objective data.

Pharmacists starting their transformation into pharmaceutical care providers should not be unduly concerned about whether medication histories, compliance data, or laboratory values are subjective or objective. The more important lesson to learn is the type of data to collect. For the sake of simplicity, many practitioners consistently consider medication histories and compliance data to be subjective, and lab tests to be objective, regardless of the source.

THE THERAPEUTIC RELATIONSHIP

The "therapeutic relationship," a cornerstone of pharmaceutical care, is a shared responsibility between the patient and the pharmacist, who agree to work together to bring about the best results possible from drug therapy. Simply put, without a therapeutic relationship, none of the steps necessary to provide pharmaceutical care can occur.

Pharmacists must gather directly from the patient most of the information needed to provide pharmaceutical care—a difficult feat without the patient's permission and cooperation. Pharmacists may wonder, Why would patients *not* want to share information that the pharmacist needs to help them? Answering this question means viewing the situation from the patient's perspective.

SUBJECTIVE AND OBJECTIVE DATA

Pharmaceutical care practitioners collect two types of data to help them evaluate and manage patients' drug therapy: subjective and objective.

- Subjective data cannot be measured directly and may not always be accurate or reproducible. Most of the data that the pharmacist collects directly from patients, such as medical history, are subjective.

- Objective data are measurable and observable, and are not influenced by emotion or prejudice. Much objective information is numerical.

Historically, pharmacists and patients have had a cordial business relationship more often than a health care relationship. And the wide variety of general merchandise for sale in many community pharmacies suggests a retail environment, not a health care setting. Most likely, the majority of a pharmacist's clientele considers her not to be in the business of health care, but rather in the business of retailing. When seen this way, it's easy to understand why patients would no more share the details of their illnesses with the pharmacist than they would with the butcher.

In a therapeutic relationship, patients recognize that the pharmacist is a health care provider and are willing to share information that they may view as private or potentially damaging. To develop such a relationship, pharmacists must demonstrate care, compassion, and discretion—and must be aware that much of what they are doing will seem foreign to most patients.

A good way to initiate the therapeutic relationship and introduce the concept of the patient interview is to say something like this: "At this pharmacy we do things a little differently. For me to help you the best I can, I need to ask you some questions that you may not have been asked before by a pharmacist. I appreciate that some of this may be rather new, but please rest assured that this information is completely confidential and will only be used to help us both make decisions about your health care."

Therapeutic relationships tend to develop slowly—sometimes over the course of months. It is important to remember that demonstrating caring will be the most valuable tool to develop this relationship. Patience will be rewarded.

THE PATIENT INTERVIEW

The patient interview is critical because it provides the pharmacist with necessary information on which to base drug therapy decisions and develop a care plan. Through the interview, the following subjective and objective data are collected:

- Demographic information, including patients' financial and insurance status;
- General health and activity status, including diet, exercise, and social information;
- Medical history;
- Medication history;
- History of present illness;
- Patients' thoughts or feelings and perceptions of their condition or disease.

The information must be timely, accurate, and complete; organized and recorded to assure that it is readily retrievable; updated as necessary; and maintained in a confidential manner. Most information can be gathered simply by talking with and observing the patient, but the interview should be organized and professional to accomplish what is intended and maximize the time spent. The interview must be confidential and private, and should be long enough to ensure that questions and answers can be fully developed without either party feeling hurried or uncomfortable.

Although much of the time pharmaceutical care practitioners will gather a more narrowly focused patient history, this chapter teaches how to take a complete history starting from basic demographic information and moving forward. The ability to gather a complete history is a critical skill, especially when a

WHICH PATIENTS SHOULD BE INTERVIEWED?

When pharmacists want to move into pharmaceutical care and start interviewing their patients, they are immediately faced with a dilemma: Whom should they interview? Who may safely not be interviewed? Often, there is no good way to tell. Consider the situation these practitioners are in. They know that drug therapy problems are ubiquitous, yet they also recognize that without interviewing patients and gathering more data, they will only do a partial job of patient care because many drug therapy problems are not immediately apparent. Pharmacist after pharmacist has found this to be a difficult issue to resolve. Although a purist might state that all patients deserve an interview, in reality there will never be sufficient time or personnel to interview every patient who possibly has a problem. See Chapter 9, Marketing Pharmaceutical Care, for some possible solutions to determining which patients to interview.

patient is seeking pharmaceutical care services but does not have a particular complaint for the pharmacist to investigate. Pharmacists in office-based practices or who market their services as "medication check-ups" will frequently find themselves in this situation. They may not have any clues about where to start in helping the patient and thus must gather a very thorough history.

GOOD INTERPERSONAL INTERACTIONS IN INTERVIEWS

Successful interpersonal interactions with patients rely on two basic skills: good communication and accurate information gathering. When pharmacists employ these skills, they start to form a professional relationship with the patient.

THE NARROW HISTORY

Unquestionably, pharmacists can continue to find some prescription and drug therapy problems using the same methods they employed before they implemented pharmaceutical care. But to take it a step further, at the end of a standard medication counseling session or when supplying a refill, pharmacists often find it useful to simply ask patients how well they think their medicines are working and if they have any questions, concerns, or problems regarding their drugs. If the answer is "yes," the pharmacist can proceed with a narrowly focused data collection session based on the patient's particular misgivings. If the answer is "no," the pharmacist can proceed to the next patient. Given the time pressures that all pharmacists practice under, rapid screening methods such as these will ensure that patients get the care they need while the pharmacist renders that care as efficiently as possible.

To some, the sort of interview described in the paragraph above may appear a half-hearted attempt to provide care. However, there is clear precedent in the health care system for this approach. For example, if a physician sees a patient for the first time who complains of symptoms of a urinary tract infection, the physician will perform a work-up of the infection and only gather other data that could reasonably influence treatment selection, such as whether the patient has a history of diabetes or prostatic hypertrophy. The physician will generally not investigate other organ systems or gather extraneous data not germane to the problem at hand. If pharmacists are to be efficient care providers, they need to develop the same screening skills.

A narrowly focused initial screening interview can be useful not only to investigate and resolve a drug therapy problem, but also to help establish a therapeutic relationship with the patient. Later, the pharmacist will likely have the opportunity to offer the patient a more in-depth interview and complete the patient's history. Many times pharmacists must do patient histories in sections, over a series of interviews, either extemporaneously or by appointment. Although pharmacists may be uncomfortable at the thought of making clinical decisions in the absence of complete information, gradually expanding one's professional database over time is the most practical approach when a complete patient interview is impossible or impractical.

The first step in beginning a patient interview is to greet the patient. Introduce oneself, smile, and shake hands firmly. If necessary, explain the interviewing process to the patient honestly and directly. Communicate warmth and welcome to the patient. Establishing friendly eye contact will convey confidence and caring.

After the greeting, direct the patient to the consultation area. Be assertive in a nonthreatening way. Use statements, not questions: for example, "Please have a seat over here," instead of, "Would you like to have a seat?"

When both pharmacist and patient are comfortable in the consultation area, explain in more detail exactly what will happen during the patient interview. A brief overview of the pharmaceutical care process may be necessary to put the interview in context. In the interest of establishing a trusting relationship, the pharmacist may want to explain why patient information is needed, how it will be stored, and how it will be used in patient care.

The pharmacist should indicate how long the interview will last. Respect the patient's schedule; it's important to ensure that this is a convenient time to conduct the interview. If it isn't, schedule an appointment.

A friendly, professional tone is a must. The pharmacist's words and manner should convey that she is a health care professional collecting necessary data. She should not feel obliged to ask permission to ask questions, nor should she appear uncomfortable or embarrassed performing the interview.

Be aware of the body language of the patient and the pharmacist. At least 55% of a message is communicated through nonverbal sources, especially in unfamiliar or uncomfortable situations. Body language that indicates warmth and interest includes friendly eye contact (not staring), leaning towards the other person, and maintaining a pleasant, concerned facial expression. Signals of discomfort, fear, or anger include avoiding eye contact, turning the body away from the other person, crossing arms, or maintaining a neutral or negative facial expression.

To get the most complete answers possible, ask open-ended questions that begin with the words "who," "what," "where," "when," "why," and "how." Open-ended questions encourage higher-level, synthesized thinking and a wide range of responses. Closed-ended questions, which simply require a "yes" or "no" answer, encourage rote recall of data and a very narrow range of answers. Avoid asking questions beginning with "are," "is," "will," "would," "do," "did," and "does." For example, instead of asking a closed-ended question, such as, "Is this the only medication

TIMING, CONVENIENCE, AND APPOINTMENTS

The best time to conduct a patient interview is as soon as a problem is suspected or at the time when the patient requests the pharmacist's assistance. Unfortunately, this may not be a convenient moment for either the patient or the pharmacist. Making an appointment to interview the patient allows both parties to set aside the time required, concentrate on the problem at hand, and complete the interview without disruption. This scheduled interview can occur in the pharmacy, over the telephone, or even in the patient's home. Another option is to perform a rapid screening interview immediately and then follow up with a more extensive, scheduled interview later.

you are taking?," ask an open-ended question, such as, "What medications are you currently taking?" This way the pharmacist encourages the patient to reflect on the question, and is more likely to get an accurate answer.

Make sure that patients are given enough time to respond. Allow lulls in the conversation to let the patient think through the question, and avoid answering the question for the patient. Listening is very important. Notice vocal tones and words that indicate subjectivity, like "I guess," and "it seems to me."

Begin with broad questions, and then get more specific, to allow the patient to follow a train of thought. Sometimes, it may be necessary to prompt patients to supply more specific information about a symptom or problem.[1,2] For example:

1. Location: "Where is the symptom/problem?"
2. Quality: "What is it like?"
3. Quantity: "How severe is it?"
4. Timing: "How long or how often has it been present?"
5. Setting: "How did it happen?"
6. Modifying Factors: "What makes it better? Worse?"
7. Associated Symptoms: "What other symptoms do you have?"

In addition to these screening questions, three questions developed by the U.S. Public Health Service are useful to determine how well patients understand their drug therapy:

1. What did your physician tell you this medication was for?
2. How did your physician tell you to use this medication?
3. What did your physician tell you to expect from this medication?

Taken together, these 10 questions provide the pharmacist with considerable patient-specific information. The seven screening questions give clues about a patient's need for medication, how well the medications are working, possible adverse effects and drug interactions and their severity, possible causative factors for symptoms, and what the patient has already done to alleviate symptoms. These questions also provide the type of data that the physician will typically need to decide how to act on a pharmacist's recommendation. If the pharmacist does not have all the data supplied by these screening questions, the physician may prefer to have the pharmacist refer the patient for medical evaluation so that the data collection process can be completed to meet the physician's needs.

The three Public Health Service questions are especially useful during medication counseling sessions because they may provide evidence that a patient has a potential problem with compliance.

Although the questions above generate valuable information, they are *screening* questions only and are not an adequate substitute for a well-taken history. If patients do not complain of symptoms, the seven screening questions may be insufficient to indicate whether the patient has a drug therapy problem. Note that all 10 questions are open ended. As the pharmacist asks them and gathers data, additional follow-up questions should focus more narrowly on the possible problems identified. Eventually, closed-ended questions can be used to identify the problem positively.

TIPS FOR GOOD INTERVIEWS: A SUMMARY

1. Greet the patient, smile, make introductions, establish friendly eye contact, and shake hands firmly.

2. Explain the interviewing process while communicating warmth and welcome.

3. Direct the patient to the consultation area in an assertive, non-threatening way.

4. Introduce the interview process in more detail, including why patient information is needed, how it will be stored, and how it will be used in patient care.

5. Indicate how long the interview will last and be sure it fits the patient's schedule.

6. Use words and manner that convey professionalism.

7. Pay attention to body language throughout the interview, including eye contact, facial expressions, and body position.

8. Ask open-ended questions. Begin with more broad questions and then get more specific.

9. Give patients adequate time for responses.

10. Use good listening skills.

11. To avoid having to think about what to say while the patient is speaking, use a list of questions as a prompt.

12. Ask the patient to restate any unclear information.

13. Communicate at the appropriate educational level and avoid medical jargon.

Listening and concentrating on the patient's descriptions should be the pharmacist's main focus. Focus on the person, not the medical condition. To listen as effectively as possible, minimize environmental distractions such as noise and nearby store traffic, and pay attention to the patient's words and nonverbal cues. Common barriers to listening include thinking about what one will say after the speaker is finished speaking; trying to do two things at once, such as listen and write; jumping to conclusions; and interrupting the speaker. If necessary, use a list of questions to guide the interview, which prevents having to think about what to say while the patient is speaking. (But remember that this is an interpersonal interaction—focus on the patient, not the form.) If necessary, tape record the interview so as not to get caught in the "note-taking rather than listening" trap. Practice focusing on the patient's actual communication instead of forecasting the patient's response and interrupting.

> **COMMUNICATION TIP:**
> **INSURMOUNTABLE BARRIERS**
>
> Sometimes it may be impossible to facilitate enough communication with a patient to conduct an acceptable interview. Examples include pediatric patients, some geriatric patients, some critical care patients, and patients with insurmountable language barriers. Under these circumstances, the pharmacist should work directly with the patient's parent, guardian, or principal caregiver.

To ensure that the information recorded is correct, the pharmacist should ask the patient to restate any unclear information. Also, the pharmacist should briefly restate the patient's words to make sure the meaning is preserved.

Communicating at the appropriate educational level is extremely important. Pharmacists should adapt their language level to that of the patient at hand and avoid medical terminology or jargon unless they are positive that the patient understands it. Talking over a patient's head does not encourage an open patient care relationship.

OTHER INFORMATION TO COLLECT

Pharmacists may want to compile other material to supplement information gathered from the patient interview, such as other pharmacy records, the patient's medical record or medical reports, comments from the patient's family, and input from the patient's other health care providers, such as physicians and other pharmacies. The pharmacist may also need to use physical assessment techniques, such as blood pressure monitoring or blood glucose testing, to acquire patient-specific objective information.

Using Data Collection Forms

An old medical axiom says that patients will always tell you what is wrong with them if only you ask the right questions. The same holds true for pharmaceutical care. With training, practice, and persistence, pharmacists can learn to ask the right questions.

During pharmaceutical care training programs, pharmacists practicing their skills often do the following. First they inquire about the patient's medication history. They follow this with a question about a lab test in the physician's office, a query into the patient's social history, and another question about medication. Given enough time, this approach will eventually provide the data the pharmacist needs, but it is inefficient, appears disorganized, and it confuses patients, who often have no idea what the pharmacist wants to know. As a result, some patients clam up and answer questions as narrowly as possible. Others respond with an "everything but the kitchen sink" approach and provide all manner of information, relevant and otherwise, and leave it to the pharmacist to sort out what is important. Neither is helpful to the pharmacist.

For pharmacists to get patients to share information in a useful way, they need to make it easy. Many have found data collection forms to be helpful tools for organizing their thoughts. A data collection form gathers related questions together so they may be asked at the same time. A well-designed form will include space for a pharmacist to record information related to:

- Basic patient demographics,
- Prescription and nonprescription drug use,
- Social and family history,
- Medical history,
- Complaints or symptoms that indicate how well drug therapy is working,
- Possible adverse effects or potential untreated conditions that will require the pharmacist's intervention or referral to a physician.

The most efficient way to collect the data is to have patients complete the form while waiting for their prescriptions to be filled. Even though most patients are used to filling out similar forms in the doctor's or dentist's office, the pharmacist should explain the nature of the form and why the information is being requested. Later, during the interview, the pharmacist can review the form with the patient and clarify and expand on sections that suggest a problem exists.

A problem with this approach is that it places substantial responsibility on the patient, who must read each question, understand it, and provide a complete, accurate answer. Sometimes a patient may simply circle an entire column of "no" with a single pen stroke, which the pharmacist should interpret as evidence that the patient did not read the form thoroughly—and thus the pharmacist should investigate further.

A second approach is for the pharmacist to complete the form during a formal patient interview. Although more time consuming, this approach may allow pharmacists to gather more and better information because they can ask follow-up questions as possible problems are revealed. It may also be a better approach for developing the therapeutic relationship. However, as suggested earlier in the chapter, if pharmacists focus too deeply on writing down the answers, they typically stop listening. When using a patient data collection form as part of a structured interview, the focus must remain on the patient. Otherwise, subtle clues and body language that the patient displays will be missed.

Commonly used data collection forms are shown in Figures 1, 2, and 3. The form in Figure 1 lends itself readily to being completed by the patient and then reviewed by the pharmacist. It is quite short, looks similar to other forms the patient is used to filling in, and inquires into all facets of the patient's history necessary to provide pharmaceutical care. It does not, however, allow a specific place for pharmacists to document their conclusions and thoughts about possible drug therapy problems. The patient or the pharmacist can complete the one-page Pharmaceutical Care History form (Figure 2), but the supplementary Medication History and Medical History form (Figure 3) is best completed by the pharmacist during the patient interview. This form is longer than the others and includes suggested questions regarding previous adverse effects, compliance, and the patient's ability to afford medications

Figure 4, the Pharmaceutical Care Data Sheet, is an abbreviated form that has been found to be most useful when only a brief or informal encounter is possible, or when providing pharmaceutical care to patients wishing to treat a condition with a nonprescription medication. Clearly, patients needing a nonprescription medication have a drug therapy problem by definition, or they would not be in the pharmacy; consequently, they may be ideal candidates for pharmaceutical care. This form is narrowly focused and does not suggest as many areas of data collection as the longer forms. Some pharmacists bind these forms into small pads that can be put in their lab coat pockets so they are easily accessible when patients need assistance with nonprescription medications. They can be used to gather information with which to assess the patient's problem and record the pharmacist's recommendation. If the patient's name and telephone number are also recorded on the form, it gives the pharmacist a convenient tool for follow-up care to assure that the problem has been alleviated.

Figure 1. Patient History Form

PATIENT HISTORY FORM

Name: _____ Date: _____

Mailing Address: _____
 street   city   state   zip

Social Security Number: _____ Phone: (H) _____ (W) _____

DOB: _____ Height: _____ Weight: _____ HR: _____ BP: _____

Gender: _____ Pregnancy Status: _____

Allergies: _____ Reactions: _____

Devices/Alerts: _____

PRESCRIPTION MEDICATION HISTORY						
Name/Strength	Directions	Start Date	Stop Date	Physician	Purpose	Effectiveness

NONPRESCRIPTION USE: Check conditions for which you have used a nonprescription medication.

____headache   ____drowsiness   ____heartburn/GI upset/gas
____eye/ear problems   ____weight loss   ____vitamins
____cold/flu   ____diarrhea   ____herbal products
____allergies   ____hemorrhoids   ____organic products
____sinus   ____muscle/joint pain   ____other: _____
____cough   ____rash/itching/dry skin
____sleeplessness

NONPRESCRIPTION MEDICATION HISTORY				
Name/Strength	Directions	Purpose	How Often	Effectiveness

FIGURE 1. PATIENT HISTORY FORM   CONTINUED

MEDICAL PROBLEMS: Have you experienced, or do you have: (circle Y or N)

known kidney problems?	Y	N		sores on legs or feet?	Y	N
frequent urinary infections?	Y	N		known blood clot problems?	Y	N
difficulty with urination?	Y	N		leg pain or swelling?	Y	N
frequent urination at night?	Y	N		unusual bleeding or bruising?	Y	N
known liver problems/hepatitis?	Y	N		anemia?	Y	N
trouble eating certain foods?	Y	N		thyroid problems?	Y	N
nausea or vomiting?	Y	N		known hormone problems?	Y	N
constipation or diarrhea?	Y	N		arthritis or joint problems?	Y	N
bloody or black bowel movements?	Y	N		muscle cramps or weakness?	Y	N
abdominal pain or cramps?	Y	N		memory problems?	Y	N
frequent heartburn/indigestion?	Y	N		dizziness?	Y	N
stomach ulcers in the past?	Y	N		hearing or visual problems?	Y	N
shortness of breath?	Y	N		frequent headaches?	Y	N
coughing up phlegm or blood?	Y	N		rash or hives?	Y	N
chest pain or tightness?	Y	N		change in appetite/taste?	Y	N
fainting spells or passing out?	Y	N		walking/balance problems?	Y	N
thumping or racing heart?	Y	N		other problems? _____	Y	N

MEDICAL HISTORY: Have you or any blood relative had: (mark all that apply)

	self	relative		self	relative
high blood pressure	___	___	heart disease	___	___
asthma	___	___	stroke	___	___
cancer	___	___	kidney disease	___	___
depression	___	___	mental illness	___	___
lung disease	___	___	substance abuse	___	___
diabetes	___	___	other _____	___	___

SOCIAL HISTORY: Please indicate your tobacco, alcohol, caffeine and dietary habits.

Nicotine Use
_____never smoked
_____packs per day for _____ years
_____stopped _____ year(s) ago

Caffeine Intake
_____never consumed
_____drinks per day
_____stopped _____ years(s) ago

Alcohol Consumption
_____never consumed
_____drinks per day/week
_____stopped _____ year(s) ago

Diet Restrictions/Patterns
_____number of meals per day
_____food restrictions: _____
_____

OTHER INFORMATION/COMMENTS:

FIGURE 2. PHARMACEUTICAL CARE HISTORY FORM

Pharmaceutical Care History

Name: _____ **Date:** _____

Allergies: (include medicines and foods) _____
_____

Unwanted Medicine Effects in the Past: _____
_____
_____

Smoking History: _____ never smoked   _____ stopped smoking
_____ packs per day for _____ years

Alcohol History: _____ never drank   _____ stopped drinking
_____ drinks per day for _____ years

Other drug use: (caffeine, marijuana etc.) _____
_____

How many meals do you eat each day? _____
What special food or diet restriction do you have? _____
Height: _____ **Weight:** _____

Family History:
Have you or any blood relative had: (mark all that apply)

	self	relative		self	relative
alcoholism	___	___	stroke	___	___
asthma	___	___	high blood pressure	___	___
cancer	___	___	kidney disease	___	___
depression	___	___	mental illness	___	___
diabetes	___	___	other conditions _____		
heart disease	___	___	_____		
lung disease	___	___	_____		

Present Medical Problems:
Have you experienced, or do you have: (circle Y or N)

known kidney problems?	Y N	sores on legs or feet?	Y N
frequent urinary infections?	Y N	known blood clot problems?	Y N
difficulty with urination?	Y N	leg pain or swelling?	Y N
frequent urination at night?	Y N	unusual bleeding or bruising?	Y N
known liver problems/hepatitis?	Y N	anemia?	Y N
trouble eating certain foods?	Y N	thyroid problems?	Y N
nausea or vomiting?	Y N	known hormone problems?	Y N
constipation or diarrhea?	Y N	arthritis or joint pain?	Y N
bloody or black bowel movements?	Y N	muscle cramps or weakness?	Y N
abdominal pain or cramps?	Y N	memory problems?	Y N
frequent heartburn/indigestion?	Y N	dizziness?	Y N
stomach ulcers in the past?	Y N	hearing or visual problems?	Y N
shortness of breath?	Y N	frequent headaches?	Y N
coughing up of phlegm or blood?	Y N	rash or hives?	Y N
chest pain or tightness?	Y N	change in appetite/taste?	Y N
fainting spells or passing out?	Y N	walking or balance problems?	Y N
thumping or racing heart?	Y N	other problems? _____	

All information is confidential. Thank you for completing this form. We will use it to better care for you.

FIGURE 3. MEDICATION HISTORY AND MEDICAL HISTORY FORM

Medication History and Medical History

Name _____ Sex _____ Birth Date _____ Ht _____ Wt _____ LBW _____ Race _____

I. Data Collection   Interview Start: _____ Stop: _____

Collected By: _____ Date: _____

Prescribed Medications

Name/Strength	Dose	Duration	Purpose	Efficacy	ADRs	Dr.	Comment

Prescribed Medications Not Currently Taking or Historical Medications

Dose/Strength	Dose	Duration	Purpose	Dr.	Why Not Still Taking

Figure 3. Medication History and Medical History Form *CONTINUED*

History Collection Form, Page - 2 Patient Name _____

Nonprescription Medications

Name/Strength	Dose	Duration	Purpose	Efficacy	ADRs	Dr.	Comment:

Completion of nonprescription medication history

What do you take for the following conditions?
(enter on OTC list, ask follow-up questions)
  headache
  eye or ear problems
  cold/flu
  allergies
  sinus
  cough
  sleeplessness
  drowsiness
  weight loss
  heartburn/stomach upset/gas
  constipation
  diarrhea
  hemorrhoids
  muscle or joint pain
  rash/itching/dry skin/skin problems

  vitamins/minerals
  herbal products/home remedies/health food store products
  natural/organic products
  other
  caffeine
  alcohol
  tobacco
  illicit drugs

FIGURE 3. MEDICATION HISTORY AND MEDICAL HISTORY FORM   *CONTINUED*

History Collection Form, Page - 3 Patient Name _____

What medication allergies do you have?
(drug name, type of reaction)

What environmental allergies do you have?

What type of adverse (bad) reactions have you had to medications in the past?

Compliance assessment
Base questions on history obtained to this point.
Your medication regimen sounds complex and must be hard to follow; how often would you estimate that you miss a dose? Everyone has problems with following a medication regimen exactly as written. What are the problems you are having with your regimen?

Payment/Reimbursement Issues
How much of a problem are medication/treatment costs?

Completion of Medical History

What other diagnoses (conditions) do you have that we haven't already covered?

Diagnosis	Onset Date	Comments

Which problems are currently active, or still a problem for you?

Pertinent ROS

Figure 4. Pharmaceutical Care Data Sheet

<u>Pharmaceutical Care Data Sheet</u>

Date: _____   R.Ph. _____
Pt. Name _____   Allergies _____

_____   _____

Medications: Diagnoses:

_____   _____
_____   _____
_____   _____
_____   _____
_____   _____
_____   _____
_____   _____

Drug Therapy Problems:

_____ _____
_____ _____
_____ _____
_____ _____
_____ _____

Notes:

_____
_____
_____
_____
_____
_____
_____
_____
_____
_____
_____
_____
_____
_____

Follow-up: _____   Recorded: _____

FIGURE 5. AUTHORIZATION TO RELEASE MEDICAL INFORMATION FORM

1 Authorization To Release Medical Information

Date_____   Name: _____

2   Date of Birth: _____

SS No.:_____   3

Address: _____

Record Number: _____

I, the undersigned, do hereby grant permission for the above named pharmacy to obtain from, release to:

_____

(Name of Person or Institution)   4

_____

(Address)

the following information from the patient's clinical record:

_____

_____   5

_____

I understand that this information will be used for the purpose of:
☐ providing information to allow pharmaceutical care to be provided to the patient.
☐ providing information to the physician regarding the care provided by the pharmacist.
☐ supporting the payment of an insurance claim.
☐ other _____

_____   6

This authorization will be valid for the period of twelve months unless otherwise specified below.   7
Release authorized for _____ days   months (circle one)

I understand that I may revoke this consent at any time by sending a written notice to the above named pharmacy. I understand that any release which has been made prior to my revocation and which was made in reliance upon this authorization shall not constitute a breach of my rights to confidentiality. I understand that I may review the disclosed information by contacting the above named pharmacy.

_____   _____
Signature of Patient or Patient's Authorized Representative   Relationship of Authorized Representative   8

_____   _____
Date   Pharmacy Representative/Date

Specific authorization for release of information protected by state or federal law
I specifically authorize the release of data and information relating to:

☐ Substance Abuse   ☐ Mental Health

☐ AIDS/HIV-related information   9 | **PROHIBITION ON REDISCLOSURE**

_____
Signature of Patient or Patient's Authorized Representative/Date

In order for the above information to released, you must sign here and above.

☐ Release mailed or information sent   10

_____
Signature/Date

Original - Pharmacy / Copy - Patient
8/2/95

PROHIBITION ON REDISCLOSURE

This form does not authorize redisclosure of medical information beyond the limits of this consent. Where information has been disclosed from records protected by federal law for alcohol/drug abuse records, by state law for mental health records or HIV/AIDS related records, federal requirements (42 CFR Part 2) and state requirements (Iowa Code chs. 228/141) prohibit further disclosure without the specific written consent of the patient, or as otherwise permitted by such law and/or regulations. A general authorization for the release of medical or other information is not sufficient for these purposes. Civil and/or criminal penalties may attach for unauthorized disclosure of alcohol/drug abuse, mental health or HIV/AIDS information.

FIGURE 5. AUTHORIZATION TO RELEASE
MEDICAL INFORMATION FORM   *CONTINUED*

Instructions for use of "Authorization to Release Medical Information" Form

This form is intended to be used when you want to either receive information from, or release information to, other care providers. It has been reviewed by the Iowa Pharmacists Association legal counsel.

Following are suggestions for how to most appropriately use this form. Each of the numbers indicates an area of the form on the attached document.

1. Enter your pharmacy name, address, and phone number.

2. Enter the date the form was completed.

3. Enter necessary patient-identifying information. This is mainly so the receiver of the form can send you the information on the correct patient.

4. Enter name and address of the health care professional or health care facility that you will be contacting. Be sure to check the box indicating whether you are gaining permission to send to, or receive from, that health care provider.

5. Enter a description of the information you are asking to receive from, or send to, the patient's health care provider. For example: vital signs, diagnosis, lab results.

6. Check the box that tells the patient or health care provider the purposes of this need for or use of information. For example: provide pharmaceutical care to the patient.

7. Enter the number of months that this release authorization will be valid, if you or the patient require it to be different than 12 months.

8. Enter signature of patient or patient representative; relationship to patient if patient representative is authorizing; date; and signature of pharmacy representative and date.

9. Check appropriate box if the information includes or requests information relating to substance abuse, mental health, or AIDS/HIV. Enter signature date and signature of patient or patient's representative. The patient or patient representative must sign and date here as well as in section 8.

10. Check box, enter signature date and signature when you send request for information, or send information to health care provider.

Although data collection forms are a valuable aid, they are best used when learning how to take a patient history. As data collection becomes easier for them, most pharmacists stop using forms because history taking becomes an ingrained skill. Pharmacists are generally advised to stop using forms as soon as is practical because they are by nature incomplete and they can interfere with the listening process. Forms are not an adequate substitute for a caring pharmacist asking questions and focusing closely on the answers.

PATIENT INFORMATION RELEASE FORM

Most of the information that pharmacists collect, either with or without a data collection form, is subjective. Although some objective information can be gathered in the pharmacy, such as lipid profiles or vital signs, most objective information is not readily available to pharmacists unless they develop a method to ask for it. The source of objective data is typically the patient's physician or, sometimes, a hospital.

The first instinct of pharmacists converting to pharmaceutical care practice is to phone the physician's office and request the necessary information. In many cases, this is sufficient, especially if the relationship between the pharmacist and physician has historically been one of mutual assistance, cooperation, and respect. If the pharmacist is not well known to the physician, or worse, is not well respected by the physician, he or she may refuse to provide the requested information. Even when pharmacists take this as an opportunity to educate the physician about the nature of and need for pharmaceutical care, the physician may still refuse to release patient information, saying that it is confidential. In such cases, a patient information release form is a useful tool to obtain necessary data.

A release form is a legal document signed by the patient that gives the physician or hospital formal permission to release certain information to another party, such as the pharmacist. A sample of a patient release form is shown in Figure 5. This form has been reviewed by a lawyer and is legal for use in the state of Iowa. Pharmacists interested in using a release form are urged to contact qualified legal sources in their own states to ensure that the form they intend to use is legally binding.

When using a release form, pharmacists must be sure to request only the information they absolutely require, such as the results of specific laboratory tests or other investigations. Poorly worded requests for "all information" will likely be returned to the pharmacist for clarification. When contacting a hospital, it is often useful to request only a copy of the admission history and physical and the discharge summary. These are fairly brief documents that succinctly summarize the patient's stay in the hospital. Requests for entire charts may result in the hospital for-warding a 350-page document as well as a bill for photocopy and other preparation costs.

It is important to send the form to the person or department that created the data desired. For instance, a laboratory test result should be requested from the lab that performed the test, not the doctor who ordered it. This will help avoid unnecessary conflicts in the release of patient information. If in doubt, the medical records department should be able to provide guidance as to the appropriate contact person or department.

SPECIFIC DATA TO COLLECT

This section provides an exhaustive discussion of the specific data elements that are included in a comprehensive patient history. In prac-tice, however, it is rarely necessary or possible to ask for every data ele-ment listed here. Pharmacists must learn to edit their questioning and focus on the areas most likely to result in relevant information.

Before gathering a specific point of data, pharmacists should reflect on how that information will help them assist the patient. If the answer is not apparent, the question should probably not be asked. For example, questions related to substance abuse may be useful to a pharmacist caring for a patient taking disulfiram, but are less likely to be asked of a patient who only drinks occasionally.

In practice, pharmacists will usually gather focused information. At minimum, the history should include the patient's basic demographics, abbreviated social history, medication and disease state histories, and a summary of the present illness. A comprehensive history should include an in-depth summary of the data elements described below.

DEMOGRAPHIC DATA

The patient's name, address, home and work telephone numbers, the best time to call, birth date (not age), gender, ethnicity, height, and weight are key demographic data to gather. Because patients may find some of these questions potentially offensive, pharmacists may wish to indicate why the information is needed. For example, African-Americans and Asian-Americans may metabolize medication at a different rate than Caucasians. When patients are not comfortable sharing their height and weight, pharmacists should indicate an estimate.

GENERAL APPEARANCE AND HEALTH STATUS

Useful information in this category includes patients' overall appearance and affect, diet, exercise and sleep habits, if they are pregnant (include due date) or breast-feeding, and if they use any medical aids or devices such as contact lenses or glucose meters.

SOCIAL HISTORY

This information, which includes the patient's occupation, economic and insurance status, and tobacco, alcohol, and caffeine use, helps the pharmacist assess how well a patient will be able to comply with a potential care plan. If a pharmacist does not appreciate the circumstances under which a patient lives, she may devise a care plan that the patient is unable to follow. For example, recommending a topical dosage form to be applied to the feet of an airline pilot who must be in the cockpit for hours at a time is doomed to failure because the patient simply cannot comply.

Social history also provides clues about the patient's living arrangements that are useful in deciding if a care plan is likely to be successful. If a woman works nights and has difficulty sleeping during the day because she has young children at home, recommending pseudoephedrine may not be wise.

In collecting information on caffeine use, remember that soft drinks, tea, and chocolate are also forms of caffeine. On occasion it may be necessary to get information on illicit drug use and sexual history, but such circumstances are rare. Questions related to these topics, and alcohol use as well, may be poorly received by the patient unless pharmacists first indicate why they need the information and what they will do with it.

When gathering a social history, pharmacists must remember that this will be very new for most patients and they may not view the pharmacist as a health care provider who needs this type of information to do her job. Pharmacists must demonstrate caring and compassion to develop the sort of relationship with a patient that permits them to gather this type of information, and must also respect the wishes of patients who choose not to supply this type of data.

MEDICATION HISTORY

Medication history forms one of two central portions of the pharmacist's patient database. A thorough medication history must include significantly more than a simple list of drugs that the patient is taking. The pharmacist should determine all agents that the patient is taking and, if appropriate, has taken in the past, including prescription drugs, nonprescription medications, physician samples, and herbal and nutritional agents. The dose, dosage form, route of administration, duration of therapy, and indication for each drug must also be obtained. Most practitioners realize that patients may get prescriptions filled at several pharmacies and therefore they inquire about medications obtained from all sources, including mail order. Be aware that patients may also borrow medications from family members or friends. Inquiries about medication sources must be made carefully so patients do not perceive them as a sales ploy to convince them to transfer all their prescriptions to a particular pharmacy.

Once the listing of relevant drugs has been obtained, the pharmacist may investigate exactly how the patient takes the medication while at home. For example, if a medication is labeled to be taken three times per day, did the patient take the medication with meals, every eight hours, or according to some other schedule? Pharmacists should also investigate the patient's compliance with therapy. Compliance questions should be asked in a nonjudgmental fashion to avoid giving the sense that the pharmacist disapproves of the patient's actions. It may be optimal to give the patient "permission" to miss doses occasionally by using such phrases as, "People often find it difficult to remember to take all their medication. How often do you think you may forget to take a dose?" Finally, storage conditions for medications should also be assessed.

The next step is to assess the patient's response to each medication, using both subjective and objective data. Subjective responses are determined by asking questions that require patients to describe what they feel the drug's effect has been on them. Such effects may be either therapeutic or adverse. Pharmacists must learn how to mix open- and closed-ended questions appropriately to gather this type of data. Initial questions should generally be open ended, such as, "How has your erythromycin been working for you?" The answers should allow the pharmacist to ask narrower follow-up questions, which may be closed ended, such as, "Have you noticed any stomach upset from your erythromycin?"

COMMUNICATION TIP: PROCEED CAUTIOUSLY

Pharmacists should pay particular attention to the exact words and phrases they use when gathering disease state histories. Although patients generally accept that a pharmacist is entitled to information about their drug therapy, few have had pharmacists ask about their illnesses in other than a cursory fashion. Proceed slowly when gathering disease state histories, ensure that patients are comfortable with your questions, and help them understand how this information will ultimately be used to help them. And before proceeding, be sure that a therapeutic relationship is under development.

Not all drugs, such as cholesterol-lowering agents, have a readily identifiable subjective therapeutic response for the patient to describe. In these cases, pharmacists must determine which objective data will allow them to assess therapeutic effect. Similarly, not all adverse effects will lead to subjective patient complaints, such as hyperglycemia caused by thiazides, so objective data may be required.

MEDICAL HISTORY

Medical history, also known as disease state history, is the other major grouping of information the pharmacist needs. Lack of adequate knowledge about a patient's medical conditions is an important factor in preventing the pharmacist from providing pharmaceutical care. It is difficult to assess if a patient is receiving the best medication when the pharmacist is uncertain of the disease a patient is taking a medication for or the status of a disease.

As with the medication history, an adequate disease state history is more than a list of diseases. Using an appropriate mixture of open- and closed-ended questions, as well as subjective and objective data, the pharmacist must determine which disease states the patient is suffering from and which, if any, medications are being used to treat them.

Potential sources of both subjective and objective data must be considered. Sometimes objective data may be generated in the pharmacy to assess the patient's disease states, such as vital signs, peak expiratory flow rates, blood sugars, serum lipid profiles, and coagulation parameters. Other data will have to come from the physician's office or hospital; pharmacists will need to determine whether a release form is necessary.

In this portion of the information-gathering phase, the pharmacist may perform a modified review of systems (ROS), in which each organ system and the effect of drugs and diseases on that organ system, and vice versa, are reviewed The ROS will be discussed in more detail in the next chapter. A complete ROS is typically neither necessary nor possible. Pharmacists must learn how to focus their review and determine which organ systems must be evaluated and which may be safely ignored in a given patient. For example, inquiries into the vision of a diabetic are well advised, since diabetics commonly have visual problems, but the eyes are not usually an organ system involved in patients with depression who are taking fluoxetine, which only rarely causes visual disturbances. Since most pharmacists are not trained to perform a physical examination, they need to learn to modify a physician's review by asking the patient questions that provide information on an organ system's level of functioning. Some pharmacists have referred to this as "jungle medicine" and find that it forces them to home in on what is both important and able to be accomplished in the community pharmacy setting.

Additional subjective information that is relevant includes patients' perceptions about which of their conditions have the greatest impact on quality of life. The pharmacist should also assess which diseases are currently stable, which are improving, and which are worsening. Finally, it is important to inquire into how well patients understand their disease states and the degree of insight that they have about their care. Such information helps pharmacists prioritize their activities when developing a care plan.

CASE STUDY

Below is the pharmacist's interview with Mary Blythe, who was introduced in the last chapter. Take special note of three key concepts illustrated by this interview:
1. The interview is organized; related questions are asked together.
2. The pharmacist uses the interview as an opportunity to educate the patient about pharmaceutical care and to market it directly to the patient.
3. The pharmacist employs the seven screening questions to evaluate Mary's symptoms.

This interview assumes that the pharmacist has already collected routine demographic and insurance information. The pharmacist has just completed routine medication counseling on Mary's new Serzone prescription and is confident that Mary understands how to take her Serzone. The pharmacist now intends to evaluate whether she is a possible candidate for a pharmaceutical care interview and work-up. If she is, the pharmacist intends to perform a comprehensive interview and explore all of Mary's conditions and medications.

Pharm: *Before letting you go, Mary, I just wanted to ask you one more question. We try to do things a little differently in this pharmacy and make absolutely sure that all your medicines are doing what they are supposed to and that all your medical conditions are being treated to your satisfaction. What problems, questions, or concerns do you have about any of your medications or medical conditions?*

MB: *In general, I feel pretty good. However, my allergies are really bothering me and I can't always breathe very well.*

Pharm: *If that's the case, do you have a bit of time so that I could ask you some questions? I need to know a little more about you and the medications you take so that I can help you as best as I can. Perhaps there is something I can do that will help you breathe better. It will only take about 10 minutes.*

CASE STUDY

MB: I guess I have a few minutes. Is this going to cost anything?

Pharm: The initial interview is free of charge. If everything checks out okay, then we're done. If there are things that I can do to help you with your medications, then there is a charge for those services as shown here in our brochure.

MB: That seems fine. I'm really unhappy about my breathing so maybe you can help. What do you need to know?

Pharm: The first thing I need to know is all the medications you are on. Most people get their prescriptions from a number of different pharmacies so I cannot always tell what medications people take from the prescriptions I fill. Have you taken Serzone before?

MB: Yes, I've been taking it for several months

Pharm: What other prescriptions do you get filled?

MB: I also have an inhaler for my allergies. It's the Vancenase AQ.

Pharm: Are there any other prescription medications you take?

MB: No, that's it.

Pharm: How about samples from the doctor, mail-order prescriptions, or medicines you might occasionally borrow from a friend or family member?

MB: No, there are none of those.

Pharm: Okay. I also need to know about any nonprescription medications you take. What do you take, say, for a headache or a cold, and what vitamins or herbal products do you take?

MB: I sometimes take Tylenol for a headache. I rarely get colds and things like that.

Pharm: Are you taking any nonprescription medicines for your allergies?

MB: Yes I am. I take Benadryl every night before I go to bed and I use Afrin Spray.

Pharm: Okay. Now that I know what medications you take, I need to know how you take them.

MB: I take my Serzone tablets twice a day, in the morning and at dinnertime. I'm supposed to use two squirts of the Vancenase in each nostril twice daily, but I only use it when I really am having trouble breathing. Like I said, I take Benadryl every night and use Afrin a couple times a day. The Tylenol I take about once a month.

Pharm: How much of the Afrin and Benadryl do you use?

CASE STUDY

MB: I take four Benadryl capsules at bedtime and a couple of sprays of Afrin in each nostril twice a day.

Pharm: Every day? For how long?

MB: Yes. I guess I have been taking them for a few months now.

Pharm: Most people find it hard to remember to take their medications exactly as prescribed. How often do you forget to take your Serzone or Vancenase?

MB: I never forget my Serzone. I set it out with my breakfast and dinner every day. The Vancenase I only take when I'm really congested, like I said.

Pharm: Why do you only take the Vancenase when you're really congested? Has the doctor or pharmacist ever told you that it works best if you take it every day?

MB: Yes, the doctor told me to use it every day, but I don't think it works very well at all. It never seems to help me.

Pharm: Okay. So the Vancenase hasn't been helping much. You told me you have taken Serzone before. How has it worked for you?

MB: I've been on it for about three months. It's been a life saver. I used to cry all the time and feel really awful. The Serzone has really helped.

Pharm: What side effects or other problems has it caused for you?

MB: None that I know of.

Pharm: No headache, upset stomach, drowsiness?

MB: No.

Pharm: One last question on your medicines. Where do you store them?

MB: On my dresser in the bedroom.

Pharm: Okay. Now I need to know a bit about the medical conditions that you have. What things are you seeing a doctor or taking medications for?

MB: I've had depression for about a year. And there are my allergies. I guess that's about it.

Pharm: Can I assume that you take the Serzone for your depression and the Vancenase, Afrin, and Benadryl for your allergies?

MB: Yes.

Pharm: Is there anything that's bothering you that you don't see the doctor about?

MB: I also have trouble sleeping. The Benadryl seems to help with that too.

CASE STUDY

Pharm: How well have you been managing with your depression and allergies lately? Are they getting better, worse, or staying about the same?

MB: My depression is much better now that I'm on Serzone. I'm back at work and doing fine. Like I said though, my allergies are killing me.

Pharm: What are you allergic to?

MB: Just about everything—dogs, cats, dust, grasses, pollens.

Pharm: Where are your allergic symptoms located?

MB: Mostly in my nose and sinuses.

Pharm: What are they like?

MB: A lot of congestion and trouble breathing but not much mucous.

Pharm: How bad are they?

MB: They bother me just about every day.

Pharm: How long have your allergies bothered you?

MB: I've been allergic for years but they weren't too bad until I moved here last year. I haven't breathed right in months.

Pharm: Is it worse at particular times or in certain locations?

MB: No, they bother me all the time.

Pharm: Have you noticed that anything makes them better or worse? What else have you tried, such as allergy shots or other medications?

MB: The Afrin does help a bit and I think the Benadryl does too. I've never tried shots.

Pharm: One last question about your medical conditions. What other symptoms or problems do you have?

MB: Sometimes I feel a bit dizzy—especially when I stand up.

Pharm: Let's check your blood pressure. (Does so.) 90/60 and your heart rate is 78. What's your usual blood pressure in the doctor's office?

MB: It's about 110/70 most of the time.

Pharm: Okay. Now I need to ask you a few questions about your lifestyle. I appreciate that these are not questions that you typically discuss with a pharmacist, but they will help me to come up with a way to assist you that will fit with the way you live.

MB: Okay. What do you need to know?

Pharm: Can you tell me if you smoke?

CASE STUDY

MB: I quit two years ago.

Pharm: Most people have an occasional cocktail. How much alcohol do you drink?

MB: I don't drink. My father was an alcoholic and I swore that would never happen to me.

Pharm: How much coffee, tea, or soda containing caffeine do you drink?

MB: I drink four or five cups of coffee a day, but I try to drink mostly decaf.

Pharm: You say you have trouble sleeping?

MB: Yes. I think it's still a bit of a symptom from my depression.

Pharm: How often do you exercise?

MB: I go for a 30-minute walk with my husband most nights after dinner.

Pharm: Okay, Mary. That's about all I need to know. It seems to me that your major issue is your allergies and that you need help with that more than your depression. If there is one thing I could do to make you feel your best, what would that be?

MB: Help me breathe better. Other than that, I'm in pretty good shape.

Pharm: The next step is for me to spend a bit of time with my books looking up your drugs and conditions to see if there is anything I can do to help. If it's okay with you, I will call you at home tomorrow night after 6 p.m. to talk over a plan for how to help you. Is that okay?

MB: That's fine. I'll look forward to your call. Thanks very much for your help.

REFERENCES

1. Boyce RW, Herrier RN. Obtaining and using patient data. *Am Pharm.* 1991;NS31:517-23.

2. de Bittner MR, Michocki R. Establishing a pharmaceutical care database. *J Am Pharm Assoc.* 1996;NS36:60-9.

Chapter 4
◆
Patient Data Evaluation

After interviewing the patient and collecting subjective and objective information, the pharmacist is still at the entry point to the Care Cycle, illustrated in Chapter 2. What must be done now is to assess the information to determine whether the patient is, in fact, suffering from drug therapy problems that must be acted on. In other words, as the Care Cycle suggests, why do anything? This chapter reviews in detail how to evaluate patients and their drug therapy.

SYSTEMATIC APPROACH IS KEY

As with collecting patient data, it is best to use a systematic, reproducible method for evaluation. A casual or careless approach will result in either identifying problems incorrectly or not finding all the problems present. To a practitioner who is just beginning the transformation into a pharmaceutical care provider, the number of steps and concepts presented here may, at first, appear daunting. How can a pharmacist manage all these questions and concerns at once? The good news is that drug therapy evaluation is not nearly as complicated as it seems initially. In this chapter the beginner is walked through the process step by step to demonstrate the entire thought process. Very few patients need to have all these issues evaluated. Experts learn to edit the process and move through it faster, so it takes a few minutes at most. Eventually it becomes an automatic process. Typically, the most time-consuming part is reading about a drug or a disease when the pharmacist does not fully understand the data collected.

Although the data gathering and data evaluation steps have been described separately in this book for teaching purposes, in reality they occur almost simultaneously. As pharmacists accumulate facts from the patient interview, they assess the information and identify drug therapy problems at the same time.

In Chapter 2, it was noted that drug therapy problems are derived from five patient needs for drug therapy: appropriate indication, effectiveness, safety, compliance, and untreated indications. Looking for opportunities to improve areas related to these needs and ensure that these needs are met is the basis of the pharmacist's evaluation.

Following a systematic method, pharmacists are able to look at these needs and pinpoint actual drug therapy problems, identify potential problems, or discover if they must gather more information. Although it is reasonable to assume that pharmaceutical care practitioners use a series of standardized questions to examine each patient need, they do not approach data evaluation this way. Instead, the typical method—illustrated in this chapter—focuses on the patient's drugs and diseases as a way to assess needs and identify problems. For a concise listing of the drug therapy problems associated with specific drug-related needs, which this chapter discusses, see Chapter 2, Table 1 (page 20).

COMPARING PROBLEMS, TREATMENTS

After determining all the patient's medical conditions, symptoms, and drug therapies, the pharmacist must compare the patient's medical problem and medication lists. The pharmacist needs to answer two basic questions:

- Are all conditions being managed?
- Are all drug therapies managing a condition?

First, the pharmacist must determine what is being done to manage each of the patient's medical conditions and symptoms. In many cases, the patient will be taking one or more medications for each condition, but it is important to note that some conditions are managed by methods other than drug therapy.

Among common nondrug therapies are diet, exercise, and surgery. Diet and exercise, especially, are therapeutic mainstays for patients with diabetes, hypertension, and other chronic conditions. An additional nondrug therapy, known as "watchful waiting," is a form of intensive patient monitoring. Physicians commonly use it when the benefits of starting drug therapy may not outweigh the risks. Patients with certain cardiac dysrhythmias, such as premature ventricular contractions, or patients who may be developing hypertension, are frequently managed this way. Until the disease is severe enough to place the patient at risk, the physician may simply elect to re-evaluate the patient at frequent intervals. Once the disease has progressed to the point where the risks of drug therapy are acceptable, as compared to the risks of untreated disease, appropriate medications can be prescribed. Watchful waiting is not the same as doing nothing. The intention is to carefully monitor the patient and only institute therapy when clearly indicated. Doing nothing would suggest that the physician had determined that therapy would be unlikely to be indicated, ever.

UNTREATED INDICATIONS

If the pharmacist establishes that a disease is not being managed by either drug or nondrug therapy, then he can conclude that the patient's need of "untreated indications" is not being met. On the other hand, if one or more symptoms are not being treated, he cannot necessarily conclude that the patient has a drug therapy problem. Only after the symptom has been evaluated, and is determined not to have been caused by a drug, can the pharmacist safely say that additional therapy may be needed and that the patient may have a drug therapy problem.

> ### QUESTIONS TO CONSIDER
>
> • Is there an untreated indication? If so, why?
>
> • Does the patient need synergistic therapy to supplement therapy already being administered?
>
> • Does the patient need prophylactic therapy?
>
> • Does each medication the patient is taking correlate with a medical condition?
>
> • Is the patient misusing medication, whether unintentionally or deliberately?
>
> • Would nondrug therapy be preferable for any of the patient's conditions?
>
> • Is the patient taking duplicate therapy without adequate cause?
>
> • Are any drugs being administered unnecessarily to treat adverse effects?

If the pharmacist determines that the patient has an untreated indication, the cause must be pinpointed. Sometimes it is because the patient has never sought medical attention. In these cases, if the patient is to be referred to the physician's care, the pharmacist must be cautious and not appear to be diagnosing a disease, which is clearly the physician's responsibility. However, the pharmacist is qualified to observe that the patient exhibits signs or symptoms consistent with a disease state, which merit medical evaluation, and that those signs or symptoms are generally managed with drug therapy. Although informing a physician of a diagnosis is inappropriate, presenting one's observations is typically much less controversial.

Another cause for an untreated condition is a need for synergistic or prophylactic therapy for the patient's condition. Patients with hypertension or an infection, for example, may need synergistic therapy to supplement the therapy already being administered. A patient with atrial fibrillation who is not being treated with an anticoagulant may need prophylactic therapy to prevent blood clots.

INDICATION FOR EACH DRUG

Once the pharmacist is satisfied that each condition is being treated (appropriateness of treatment will be considered later), the next step is to ensure that each medication is correlated with a medical condition. If the pharmacist cannot state with certainty why a patient is taking a medication, the drug therapy may not be necessary. Before automatically reaching this conclusion, however, the pharmacist should first think about whether more data are needed. Sometimes patients do not know the indication for their medications, which requires the pharmacist to confirm the indication with the physician or a family member.

Patients who were started on medication for an acute condition while they were in the hospital are particularly at risk to have no medical indication for a drug. The continuity of care between the hospital and ambulatory settings is often problematic and confusions with medications are common. Pharmacists trained in pharmaceutical care practice have reported cases where patients received laxatives or nitrates for many years after hospital discharge. Such patients were treated with drugs in the hospital to manage acute constipation or chest pain, but were never told to discontinue them, even though the conditions were resolved. The patients simply assumed that the doctor wanted them to continue; the doctor simply assumed that the patient was chronically constipated or had ongoing angina. Outside of a pharmaceutical care practice, pharmacists would not intervene since there was no apparent problem. These patients were misusing their drugs, but were doing so unintentionally.

Just as patients may misuse their medications unintentionally, so may they misuse them deliberately. Most pharmacists are already attuned to inappropriate drug-seeking behavior by patients. Because pharmaceutical care practitioners have a greater patient database available, they can verify indications for drug therapy and reach conclusions about misuse more confidently.

As pharmacists assure that each drug has an appropriate indication, they should also determine if nondrug therapy would be preferable. Such a finding is much less likely for prescribed medications, since the need for therapy has been determined by the physician, than it is for nonprescription medications. When patients attempt self-care, they typically do not try to balance the risks and benefits of drug versus nondrug therapy; the pharmacist may be able to decide if nondrug therapy is a better choice. For example, patients frequently take vitamins for "energy," a use for which they are ineffective. A pharmaceutical care provider can work with a patient to review diet, exercise, and sleep patterns and institute a nondrug therapeutic plan.

If a patient is taking duplicate therapy without adequate cause, this is also a drug therapy problem. In the past, such problems were typically identified by computer screening programs. Since these programs do not use patient-specific data, some so-called problems turned out to be a deliberate, rational use of two medications. Using a pharmaceutical care model, the pharmacist is able to determine whether duplicate therapy is rational pharmacotherapy.

COMMON NONDRUG THERAPIES

- Diet
- Exercise
- Surgery
- "Watchful waiting": intensive patient monitoring.

The final problem related to appropriateness of indication is using a drug unnecessarily to treat the adverse effects of a second drug. Patients who are on multiple medications—often the elderly—are at particular risk for this problem, which is something pharmacists may uncover as they verify the indications of a patient's medications. If the patient does not need the medication causing the adverse effect, or if it can be safely changed to another medication without the same side-effect profile, then clearly it is a case of an avoidable adverse effect. If, on the other hand, the drug causing the adverse effect cannot be changed or discontinued, then the adverse effect is not avoidable and may need to be treated.

Having completed the patient work-up thus far, the pharmacist has ensured that every medication has an indication and that every indication has a medication—or at least a therapy. In so doing, the pharmacist is now able to assess whether the patient's needs of appropriate indication and untreated indication have been met. Furthermore, the pharmacist should be able to identify any drug therapy problems related to these needs. If the pharmacist still cannot make this assessment confidently, then he needs to gather further data and repeat the evaluation.

SAFETY, EFFICACY, AND COMPLIANCE

Drug therapy problems related to safety and efficacy are among the most common areas for pharmacist-physician conflict. The best way to avoid conflicts is for the pharmacist to have adequate evidence that the patient demonstrates, or is at risk for, harm from the drug therapy problem. Such evidence absolutely requires patient-specific data.

Consider the following example: A pharmacist is about to refill a prescription for digoxin 0.25 mg, to be taken by mouth once a day, for a 77-year-old man who is transferring his prescription into the pharmacy. Using the old model of practice, the pharmacist might determine that this dosage is likely to be excessive. Therefore the patient's potential drug therapy problem would be too-high dosage, caused by the wrong dose. A phone call to the physician to discuss this potential problem may not resolve it to the pharmacist's satisfaction, since all he can do is voice his concern that, according to the literature, 0.25 mg of digoxin is a high dose in elderly patients, who often have some renal impairment. Under a pharmaceutical care model, however, the pharmacist would have gathered patient-specific data such as pulse rate. If the patient demonstrated bradycardia, the pharmacist would have much stronger information to back up his claim of excessive dosage.

When pharmacists evaluate pharmacotherapy for drug therapy problems related to safety and efficacy, they must try to use patient-specific information as often as possible. Otherwise, they are less likely to convince physicians that a problem exists.

Unlike patient needs related to indication, it is difficult to evaluate needs related to safety, efficacy, and compliance one at a time. The evaluation can still be done systematically, but the same question may cover more than one patient need. To draw valid conclusions, the pharmacist must follow an organized approach, using as much patient-specific data as possible.

First the pharmacist must review the dose, dosage interval, duration of therapy, and dosage form for each drug on the patient's medication list. Since this practice requires the pharmacist to review both the drugs themselves and the patient's response to them, it provides evidence of how well the patient's drug needs for safety and efficacy are being met.

APPROPRIATENESS OF THE DOSE

Is each drug's dose appropriate, too high, or too low? This is the first question pharmacists should ask themselves during their systematic evaluation. Judgments on the appropriateness of the medication strength should, as much as possible, be made using patient-specific data such as age, weight, concurrent drugs and diseases, pregnancy or lactation status, and so on. It is best not to depend solely on the dosing information in a reference text, unless absolutely necessary.

To definitively evaluate the appropriateness of the dose, it is necessary to assess the patient's response to the medication. If a dose is felt to be too low but subjective and/or objective data suggest that the patient is responding to the drug, it is difficult to justify a conclusion that the patient has an actual drug therapy problem of too low a dose. Similarly, if a patient does not exhibit signs or symptoms of adverse effects or toxicity, concluding that there is an actual problem of too high a dose may not be plausible.

On the other hand, potential drug therapy problems are often identified by simply determining the patient's risk. The size of this risk is usually estimated using information from the literature. For example, a patient with impaired renal function is receiving a "normal" dose of lithium carbonate for his mania. Lithium is a potentially toxic drug excreted by the kidneys. A drug information handbook suggests that the dose of lithium should be decreased by 25% to 75%, depending on the patient's kidney function. Even if this patient does not exhibit the sedation or confusion normally seen with lithium toxicity, the patient does have a potential drug therapy problem because the risks and consequences of lithium toxicity are severe.

In summary, evidence of clinical response, evidence of adverse effects, and potential risk for harm should all be considered when evaluating the appropriateness of the patient's dose.

Once satisfied that the appropriate strength of the patient's medication has been prescribed, the pharmacist can move on to consider other reasons why the dose may not be optimal. When patients store medications in an excessively hot and humid location, or if the medication is past its expiration date, the dosage form may degrade enough that the patient receives a subtherapeutic dose. Similarly, when patients administer their medication incorrectly, they may receive too high or too low a dose, even if the initial choice of dose was well made. Finally, the pharmacist should screen for any drug interactions that may result in potential or actual exposure to toxic or subtherapeutic drug levels. A drug interaction is definitively discovered if the patient exhibits clear evidence of it. If no such evidence is present, then the pharmacist should assess how likely the emergence of the interaction is and how severe its consequences may be.

Dosage Schedule

Is the dosage schedule appropriate, too frequent, or too infrequent? This question is related both to the patient's need for safe and efficacious drug therapy and to the question of whether a dosage is too high or too low.

Dosage interval is evaluated in the same fashion as dosage strength; the patient's clinical response and evidence of toxicity must be examined. If no sign of undesirable outcomes is found, the patient does not have an actual drug therapy problem. There may be a potential problem, however, which would be pinpointed in the same way as potential problems related to dosage strength.

DURATION OF THERAPY

Is the duration of each drug therapy appropriate, too long, or too short? The same issues apply as for dosage strength and interval. Patient-specific data must be evaluated, if possible, before the pharmacist concludes that an actual problem exists; literature may be used to justify the existence of a potential problem.

DOSAGE FORM

The issue of dosage form bears special mention. No other health care provider has the training in dosage forms that pharmacists have. Indeed, knowledge of dosage forms is one of pharmacists' unique talents. Pharmaceutical care providers put this knowledge to use by evaluating the appropriateness of each dosage form for their patients.

> ## QUESTIONS TO CONSIDER
>
> - Are the dose, dosage interval, duration of therapy, and dosage form appropriate for each medication the patient is taking?
>
> - Is the patient responding appropriately to the drug?
>
> - Is there evidence of adverse effects or drug allergies?
>
> - Are the medications being stored properly and are any past their expiration dates?
>
> - Are medications being administered correctly?
>
> - Are there any potential or actual drug interactions?

Problems with dosage form seem be found most commonly with inhaled medications, which the pharmacist identifies by checking a patient's technique with a metered dose or other inhaler. However, there are issues of dosage form with other routes of administration, as well. Injection technique and appropriateness of the parenteral route should be evaluated for patients self-injecting medications while at home.

Depending on the dosage form being considered, pharmacists should ask themselves a variety of questions:

- Does the patient have the visual acuity and manual dexterity to prepare a dose accurately?
- Will a topical, otic, ophthalmic, or rectal dosage form be stored and administered correctly?
- Do the patient's job or school activities prevent him from using the dosage form properly?
- If the patient is using a patch, does she understand how to apply it and how often to change it?
- Can the patient physically swallow all oral dosage forms or is he crushing them?
- Are sustained release products being used correctly?

- Are liquid dosage forms measured accurately before being administered? Are they stored correctly and shaken before use as required?

- Are sublingual products being used correctly?

THE RIGHT OR WRONG DRUG

After evaluating the dosage form, the pharmacist must ensure that each drug the patient is on is the right one for the condition.

Arguments of "right drug" versus "wrong drug" are as old as clinical pharmacy and have historically been a significant area of tension between pharmacists and physicians. As explained in Chapter 2, declaring that a patient suffers from the drug therapy problem of "wrong drug" can inadvertently offend the physician. The pharmacist-physician relationship often plays an important role in how problems related to drug therapy choice are evaluated and solved. Although each professional functions by using the skills and values unique to his or her profession, their perspectives are typically very different. Historically, the physician's primary consideration was the patient, while for the pharmacist, it was usually the drug therapy—or at least it appeared that way to the physician.

> **QUESTIONS TO CONSIDER**
>
> - Is each drug the patient is on the right one for the condition?
> - Does the patient have any clear contraindications to a drug?
> - Is the patient's condition refractory to the therapy?
> - Is more effective therapy available than the agent that the patient is on?

Pharmacists and physicians also tend to use different data to make decisions. Physicians use a combination of what they know from their reading and what they have learned from managing similar patients in the past. Since most pharmacists have historically not monitored patients in any significant sense, they tend to base their evaluations on what they have read, rather than on what they have done. The task of pharmaceutical care providers is to change this situation and demonstrate that the patient is at the center of their efforts. This is best accomplished by having a solid grasp of the patient-specific facts, a good knowledge base of drugs and diseases, and, perhaps most important, an open mind. Although disagreements are sometimes based on turf issues, they are just as likely to stem from physicians not realizing that pharmacists' motivation is patient care. Pharmacists need to help physicians understand that patient care is their mutual, primary interest.

The issue of a "wrong drug" caused by an inappropriate dosage form has already been discussed. It is also an example of a drug therapy problem for which the physician is more disposed to accept the pharmacist's judgment.

CONTRAINDICATIONS

If a patient has a clear contraindication to a drug, that, too, is a wrong choice of drug. Physicians are generally inclined to accept pharmacists' recommendations in such cases because choosing a clearly contraindicated drug opens them up to a lawsuit. Much more often, however, the contraindication is relative, not absolute. Relative contraindications are a matter of judgment, and the pharmacist and physician will not always agree on how important a relative contraindication is. As much patient-specific knowledge as possible, and a good knowledge of the literature, are the pharmacist's key tools for dealing with questions of possible contraindications.

REFRACTORY CONDITIONS OR MORE EFFECTIVE THERAPY

Another reason for deciding a drug is "wrong" is that the patient's condition is refractory to the therapy. This may be seen, for example, in patients on oral hypoglycemic therapy who have not responded to maximal doses of multiple drugs. In patients whose diabetes may have become refractory to sulfonylureas, the role of insulin needs to be explored. Or, perhaps the patient is not responding to therapy because the drug being used is not indicated for the condition. Finally, there may be more effective drug therapy available than the agent currently prescribed. These are all judgment calls. Whether a condition has become refractory can only be determined if there is convincing evidence, either subjective or objective, that the patient is no longer responding to therapy. Because this conclusion involves decisions about pathophysiology and how the disease state is progressing, physicians may view pharmacists' involvement as an attempt to diagnose or evaluate a disease state.

Determining that more effective therapy is available is a common source of interprofessional conflict. Pharmacists tend to use information they have read to decide if better drug therapy is available, whereas physicians use a combination of what they have read and what they have previously done. If a physician has had good clinical success with a given drug in a certain situation, the pharmacist may find it difficult to convince the physician that it is a poor therapeutic choice. Another scenario that can defy logical arguments about rational pharmacotherapy is when physicians select a certain drug because it is new and they want to try it in a few patients to gain experience using it.

The drug therapy problem of "wrong drug" causes great difficulty for most beginning pharmaceutical care practitioners. Pharmacists who have read this far may feel apprehensive at the thought of contacting physicians to correct problems related to choice of therapy, since the problems appear to be so controversial. But keep in mind that physicians can and *do* make errors in choosing medications. When they do, they are generally receptive to the pharmacist's opinions—especially when the opinions are phrased in a way that reflects the pharmacist's concern for the patient.

Disagreements occur most often when the drug therapy problem is not an obvious one. Rational decisions on the choice of drug therapy, as well as choices related to dose, dosage intervals, and duration of therapy, reflect both the art and science of pharmacotherapeutic decision-making. Pharmacists must realize that competent, well-intentioned professionals can and do disagree about these decisions every day. They may not agree that a problem even exists, let alone what to do about it. This does not make one party right and the other wrong; much of the time, they disagree because they have reached different conclusions from the same data. Pharmaceutical care providers learn not to be emotionally overinvested in these types of disagreements. They take them in stride and learn from them. They work hard to keep the lines of communication with the physician open so that, as less arguable problems are discovered, the physician will be receptive to the pharmacist's input.

> ## Unapproved Indications
>
> "Indication" refers to more than the federally approved indications listed in the product monograph. Physicians use drugs for nonindicated conditions all the time, most often because they have read medical literature that supports the drug's usefulness in treating the condition. Although the drug is not officially approved for a certain use, they have evidence that it may be effective, and prescribe accordingly. In other instances, physicians combine what they know of the patient's pathophysiology and the drug's pharmacology to make a considered decision that the drug is likely to be effective. Before pharmacists conclude that a drug is not indicated, it is imperative that they too consider the patient's condition and determine if there is at least a theoretical reason why the drug could work. If not, the pharmacist needs to find out if the physician is aware of information with which the pharmacist is not familiar.

Compliance Issues

Next, the pharmacist addresses the patient's need for compliance with drug therapy. Is the patient complying or not? Since most pharmacists have spent their careers assisting patients with compliance problems, this is usually firm ground. In a pharmaceutical care practice, however, identifying a compliance problem is only the first step; pharmacists must also ferret out the cause of the patient's noncompliance.

Typically, pharmacists detect noncompliance by checking refill dates against days of therapy supplied or performing actual pill counts. Pharmaceutical care practitioners will also use the patient interview as an opportunity to ask specifically how well the patient has complied with drug therapy. Most causes for inappropriate compliance can only be identified by evaluating the information gathered during the patient interview.

Occasionally, a patient cannot be compliant because the drug product is not available. It may be a new drug that is not yet in the wholesaler's catalogue, it may have been discontinued, or it may be back ordered by the manufacturer. In these cases, the pharmacist will need to work with the physician and patient to find alternative therapy.

Often, patients exhibit poor compliance because they cannot afford the cost of the drug therapy. Most pharmacists are familiar with this situation and will try, when possible, to switch the patient to a more affordable agent. Although this situation *does* represent an actual drug therapy problem, the pharmacist must carefully consider the possible disadvantages of switching therapies when developing the care plan (see Chapter 5). Changing drugs on the basis of cost alone is not always wise. In a patient whose disease is stable, and who is not exhibiting problems with adverse effects or drug interactions, changing to another agent may place the patient at risk for new problems, including loss of clinical efficacy or side effects. From the patient's perspective, citing excessive drug cost is a plausible explanation for poor compliance that may or may not be truly related to cost. Sometimes, when the patient perceives a drug cost as excessive, patient education on the nature of costs versus benefits is all that is required to remedy a compliance problem.

> ### QUESTIONS TO CONSIDER
>
> - Is the patient complying with drug therapy, and if not, why not?
> - If the patient finds a therapy too expensive, what alternatives are possible?
> - What are the possible disadvantages to switching therapy?

An inability to swallow or otherwise administer the dosage form is another cause for inappropriate compliance. Generally, pharmacists will identify this problem when they evaluate the appropriateness of the dosage form.

Patients may not comply with therapy because they do not understand what it is for or what is required of them. Asking the three Public

Health Service screening questions in Chapter 3 (see page 32) will give pharmacists ample evidence if this is the source of noncompliance.

Finally, some patients are deliberately noncompliant. They may feel that the medication is not working; they may believe it is causing more problems than it treats; they may have a different goal for therapy than the pharmacist or physician does; or they may simply not want to take the drug. Having to take a drug, especially for a chronic condition, reminds patients daily that there is something wrong with them. Simple education and reassurance may not always be enough to motivate such patients to comply with therapy. The pharmacist needs to work with them to help them see the benefits of therapy, and must be considerate of their fears and concerns. Sometimes, the underlying issue can be identified and readily addressed, but ultimately, it becomes a patient's personal decision to comply. If, despite the pharmacist's good faith effort to educate the patient, and the patient's apparent understanding, the patient still refuses drug therapy, the problem does not really exist until the patient accepts it as a problem.

> ## ULTIMATELY, COMPLIANCE IS PATIENT'S DECISION
>
> Education and reassurance may not always be enough to motivate patients to comply with drug therapy. Pharmacists must work with patients to help them see the benefits of therapy and must be considerate of their fears and concerns. Sometimes, the underlying issue can be identified and addressed, such as the medication's cost or the patient's difficulty swallowing it. Many times, however, it becomes a patient's personal decision to comply.

ADVERSE EFFECTS AND DRUG INTERACTIONS

Assessment adverse effects and drug interactions is discussed last because, as the pharmacist examines the patient's response to drug therapy in previous portions of the evaluation, most problems of this nature will be revealed without specifically looking for them. Adverse effects related to drugs not considered safe for the patient should be found when determining if the patient is on the right drug. Similarly, adverse effects caused by rapid changes in dose or improper drug administration should be found when the dose and dosage form are evaluated. The one type of adverse effect that must be identified separately is related to drug allergy. As pharmacists evaluate the patient, they must consider if any of the patient's conditions could be explained by an allergic reaction to a medication.

REVIEW OF SYSTEMS

If the pharmacist has diligently evaluated the patient's medical conditions, symptoms, and drug therapies, all the patient's drug therapy problems should be identified. The final task is to perform an evaluation of the patient as a whole, which is accomplished by a review of systems (ROS).

For physicians, the ROS is the heart of the physical examination. To the pharmaceutical care practitioner, a modified ROS acts as a quality assurance check: a final opportunity to examine whether the patient's medications are causing problems and whether the patient's organ functions will have an effect on drug therapy.

Since few pharmacists are trained to perform a physical examination, the pharmacist's ROS is more of a mental activity. It involves considering the patient's organ systems one by one and determining how each may be evaluated in the pharmacy setting. Often, pharmacists will have only limited, subjective data on which to base conclusions. Nevertheless, a modified ROS is an important step in identifying drug therapy problems.

The first area of review is readily available to the pharmacist: the patient's vital signs. The pharmacist should look into whether the

---

DISAGREEMENTS ON WHAT TO CALL A PROBLEM

As pharmacists identify various drug therapy problems, they will immediately notice that, although they and other pharmacists or physicians will generally agree on the existence of a problem, they will frequently disagree on what to call it. For example, if a patient with a history of bleeding ulcers suffers gastric pain after taking prednisone for asthma, is the problem "unsafe drug for patient," "adverse effect," "inappropriate dosage form," or something else?

Pharmacists are encouraged to identify all the possible choices for what any given problem may be and then work through each potential problem for errors in logic or interpretation of patient data or literature that suggest another choice is more rational. Even after such an exercise, however, several equally valid choices may remain. In such cases, the nature of the problem is frequently dictated by the nature of the care plan. Essentially, the exact cause of the prob-

lem is defined retrospectively. In the previous example, if taking the prednisone with an antacid is thought to be a valid recommendation, then the problem could be fairly characterized as an adverse effect or a need for additional therapy. If another pharmacist suggests that the prednisone could be safely changed to a steroid inhaler, then identifying the problem as an incorrect dosage form may be more reasonable. Although different pharmacists may never come to consensus on the strict definition of a problem, they should become comfortable in defending their conclusions based on interpretation of patient-specific and literature-based data. Pharmacists should not be overly concerned at identifying the problem "correctly" since multiple, equally correct choices are common. Rather, they should be sure that they have identified all the patient's problems, and then should develop a care plan for each.

patient's temperature, heart rate, blood pressure, or respiration rate are affected by the drug therapy and, therefore, whether they need to be closely monitored in this patient.

Since many drugs are either cleared by the liver and kidneys or may be toxic to them, pharmacists must be certain that there is no evidence of drug-induced damage to these organs. They should also attempt to verify that the metabolic functions of these organ systems have not deteriorated to the point where changes in drug dosage are needed. In patients with poor hepatic function, the accompanying effects on blood clotting and protein synthesis must be considered for drugs that affect coagulation or are highly protein bound.

The patient's fluid and electrolyte status can be briefly evaluated by assessing the patient for signs and symptoms of edema or dehydration. Cramping, fatigue, muscle weakness, or spasms may be evidence of electrolyte derangements. The effect of the patient's therapy on fluid and electrolyte status must be considered since the most common cause of alterations in this system is the use of diuretics. Conversely, edema or dehydration may affect the pharmacokinetics of many drugs and must be considered when the dose is evaluated.

The effect of drugs on the patient's cardiovascular system, and vice versa, should be taken into account. Consider whether the patient's medications could affect blood pressure, cardiac rhythm, cardiac function, or blood lipids.

Certain pulmonary diseases may contraindicate some kinds of drug therapy. For example, patients on beta blockers or estrogens should be evaluated for obstructive airway disease or a history of pulmonary embolism. The need for pulmonary monitoring in the pharmacy, such as peak expiratory flow rates, should be evaluated.

Evaluate the patient's hematological system. Evidence of altered coagulation, oxygen-carrying capacity, or infection-fighting ability will affect the use of drugs in such patients. This evaluation is especially important for patients on drugs that may cause bleeding, clotting, anemia, or immunosuppression.

The effect of drugs on the endocrine system must be monitored. Consider whether the patient's glucose control or thyroid function may be affecting drug therapy, as well as whether the drug therapy may affect the patient's blood sugar or thyroid gland.

Since diarrhea is such a common adverse effect, any changes in the function of the gastrointestinal tract must be investigated. The patient's ability to absorb oral medications should also be taken into account.

The final two organ systems that commonly have a significant influence on drug therapy are the neurological and dermatological systems. Drug therapy often causes central nervous system effects. The most common sign of drug allergies is a skin rash. The pharmacist should ascertain if any changes in the patient's nervous system or skin may be drug induced.

The remainder of the ROS considers organ systems that are less likely to be affected by drug therapy, such as the genitourinary and musculoskeletal systems; eye, ear, nose, and throat; and psychological functioning. A brief review of how these systems are performing is required to rule out drug therapy problems.

CONCLUSION

As pharmacists complete their evaluation of a patient's drug therapy, they frequently find that they would like to have more patient information before making a final determination. This is not a cause for panic. Sometimes, missing facts do not make any significant difference and the pharmacist can proceed. Other times, it is necessary for the pharmacist to contact the patient to obtain the missing information. As will be seen in the next chapter, no care plan should be implemented without first discussing it with the patient. This allows the pharmacist one last opportunity to gather the final few bits of data that were forgotten during the initial interview.

CASE STUDY

Now that the pharmacist has initiated a therapeutic relationship with Mary Blythe and gathered an extensive patient history, he has to consider the data and determine if Mary has any drug therapy problems. Note that the pharmacist has gathered much more information than will be needed to identify her drug therapy problems. Some of this data will be used later, when developing a care plan for Mary. The pharmacist begins by looking at Mary's medication list and her list of diseases and symptoms.

Mary's medications include:
- *Serzone 150 mg by mouth twice daily,*
- *Vancenase AQ 2 sprays by nasal inhalation twice daily when she has difficulty breathing,*
- *Tylenol occasionally for headache,*
- *Afrin Nasal Spray 2 sprays twice daily,*
- *Benadryl 4 capsules at bedtime.*

Mary has been taking all these medications for at least several months.

Mary's conditions and symptoms include depression, multiple environmental allergies with considerable nasal congestion, difficulty sleeping, and blood pressure of 90/60.

Comparing Mary's drugs and conditions, it appears that each drug has an acceptable indication. Serzone is medically indicated for depression, Vancenase AQ, Benadryl, and Afrin for allergies and congestion, and Tylenol for headaches. The pharmacist concludes that Mary does not have any problems caused by a lack of medical indication, there is no evidence of recreational drug use or addiction, and it does not appear that avoidable adverse effects are being treated with additional drug therapy. The role of nondrug therapy and the multiple therapies for Mary's allergies remain to be clarified to see if there are problems.

When looking at Mary's conditions and symptoms, it appears that the depression, allergies, and insomnia are being treated, but that her low blood pressure is not. It is not yet clear, however, if Mary needs additional drug therapy to treat any of her conditions.

CLINICAL AND ADVERSE RESPONSES

Mary's clinical and adverse responses to her medications are evaluated to see if further drug therapy is indicated. She feels that her depression has responded well to Serzone and she does not complain of any adverse effects that she would attribute to Serzone. Her insomnia is only partly controlled and her allergies and nasal congestion are not well controlled at all. Indeed, breathing difficulty is her major complaint. Also, her blood pressure is quite low and she is not receiving drug or nondrug therapy for it.

CASE STUDY

Before the pharmacist decides that Mary needs additional drug therapy for her complaints, however, he must determine if any of these symptoms could have been caused by drug therapy. The insomnia does not appear to be drug induced, nor does it appear to be related to excessive caffeine intake. The nasal congestion may well be due to rebound congestion caused by excessive use of Afrin over several months. The pharmacist is also aware that Serzone has alpha-adrenergic blocking properties that may be partially responsible for both Mary's congestion and low blood pressure. The pharmacist decides that Mary does not require additional drug therapy, but that additional nondrug therapy may prove helpful for her insomnia.

By now, the pharmacist is reasonably confident that all Mary's drugs carry an indication and that all her conditions that should be managed by drug therapy are being so treated. The pharmacist now moves on to consider issues related to safety, efficacy, and compliance.

SAFETY, EFFICACY

The first step is to consider the dose, dosage interval, duration of therapy, and dosage form for each of Mary's medications, beginning with the Serzone. The pharmacist knows that 300 mg per day of Serzone is at the low end of the dosing range. However, since Mary claims a good therapeutic response to her Serzone, there does not appear to be any reason to increase the dose. On the other hand, some of Mary's congestion may be caused by the Serzone, so perhaps a decrease in dose could be considered. Mary takes her Serzone twice a day, has done so for several months, and seems to have no problem taking the tablets correctly. The pharmacist concludes that there are no apparent problems with Serzone dosing.

The same process is carried out for Mary's Vancenase AQ, Benadryl, Afrin Spray, and Tylenol. A variety of problems immediately becomes apparent. The true dose of Vancenase AQ is unclear since Mary only uses it when she feels she needs to. This suggests a compliance problem and is an example of how pharmacists can find one problem while looking for another. Given Mary's complaint of poor breathing, it is clear that Mary has a problem related to her Vancenase AQ. Although poor compliance may be a factor, so may poor inhaler technique. Mary's technique was not evaluated during the interview. Now the pharmacist has to decide how to proceed without this piece of very useful information.

Mary claims to be taking four capsules of Benadryl at bedtime. This likely means she is taking 100 mg total each night, since 25 mg capsules are the most widely available over the counter. Mary is taking the equivalent of an entire day's dose

CASE STUDY

of Benadryl at one time. Although she does not have any immediately apparent evidence of adverse effects from such a large dose, the pharmacist would nevertheless conclude that this is an excessive dose. Benadryl's anticholinergic activity may be worsening Mary's breathing through excessive drying of her nasal mucosa. In addition, hypotension is reported as an uncommon side effect of Benadryl. Mary has taken Benadryl for several months and has done so, in part, as a sleep aid. This suggests that the duration of therapy may be a potential problem for Mary. Finally, there is no evidence that the dosage form is problematic here.

Mary's Afrin Nasal Spray is also found to be causing a problem. Although her inhalation technique is not clear, it is apparent that she has been using the spray for long enough to have developed symptoms consistent with rebound congestion. Even though she still complains of trouble breathing, her duration of therapy is excessive since other, safer therapy should be used for her long-term allergy control.

Mary's Tylenol is the final medication to be evaluated. The actual dose that Mary takes is not clear. This is unfortunate in a patient who has demonstrated a propensity to use medications at higher than their labeled doses. The pharmacist would be well advised to ensure that Mary's single-dose use of Tylenol is not potentially damaging to her liver. The other factors related to duration of therapy, dosage form, and dosage schedule are not problems in Mary.

The last two possible areas for dosing-related problems do not appear to be relevant for Mary. Dosing problems due to storage do not appear to be a concern since Mary keeps her medicines in a cool, dry place. Neither is there any evidence of a drug interaction resulting in a problem related to drug dosing.

CORRECT DRUGS

Having completed an evaluation of Mary's drug dosing, the pharmacist can now move on to consider if Mary is on the correct drug for each of her conditions. There are no apparent contraindications to Mary's Serzone; her depression is not refractory to it, the drug is clearly indicated for depression, no dosage-form problems exist, and there is no reason to believe that Mary should be switched to a possibly more effective drug. Therefore, the pharmacist can safely conclude that Serzone is a good choice for Mary's depression.

The same evaluation for Mary's Vancenase AQ reveals that there are no contraindications and it is indicated for her allergies. Determining if her allergies are refractory or if more effective therapy is available is difficult; Mary's lack of compliance makes it impossible to assess her response to the drug. The role of the

CASE STUDY

dosage form is not clear since the pharmacist did not verify inhaler technique during the patient interview. The pharmacist concludes that, although there are problems related to the Vancenase AQ, they are not a result of the physician's choice of drug. Evaluations of Mary's Afrin Spray, Benadryl, and Tylenol follow a similar line of reasoning. Certainly, there are problems with Mary's use of Afrin and Benadryl, but they are not a result of drug selection. There do not appear to be any problems related to the choice of Tylenol.

COMPLIANCE PROBLEMS

The pharmacist's identification of compliance problems in Mary is a rapid exercise. She has stated explicitly that each day she remembers to take her Serzone both morning and evening. As the pharmacist develops an ongoing relationship with Mary, her compliance may be verified by comparing refill dates with the days of medication supplied. Similarly, Mary seems to be completely compliant with her Afrin and Benadryl — if excessive use can be termed compliance. She claims to use the Benadryl every night and the Afrin twice daily. Since Tylenol is taken only as needed, compliance does not appear to be a problem. Mary does, however, have a compliance problem with her Vancenase AQ.

The exact cause of Mary's lack of compliance is not immediately clear. Since she claims that her physician told her it should be taken daily, the pharmacist could reasonably conclude that Mary understands the instructions. The product is readily available and Mary has prescription insurance, so lack of availability and excessive cost are ruled out. The final two causes for poor compliance are the patient's inability to administer the drug or a preference not to use it. Mary has clearly stated that she does not think Vancenase AQ works for her allergies, so it seems that her noncompliance is largely a matter of patient preference.

ADVERSE REACTIONS

Since the pharmacist's evaluation of Mary's drug therapy is largely complete, assessment of drug safety has been partially completed, as well. The pharmacist already suspects that Mary's congestion is largely due to misuse of Afrin coupled with the alpha-blocking effects of Serzone. The Serzone is also the most likely cause of Mary's low blood pressure—again, because it is an alpha blocker. The excessive dose of Benadryl may play a role in Mary's breathing if the anticholinergic, drying effects have excessively dried out her nasal mucosa; hypotension also is a reported side effect of Benadryl. Since there is no direct evidence of nasal drying, however, and since hypotension is rare, it is more likely that the Serzone and Afrin are responsible for Mary's complaints. The pharmacist concludes that Mary shows evidence of several adverse drug reactions, but there is no evidence of drug interactions.

CASE STUDY

REVIEW OF SYSTEMS

Finally, the pharmacist performs a brief review of systems. Mary's vital signs are abnormal as reflected by low blood pressure. This is attributed to the Serzone. There is no evidence to suggest that Mary has renal or hepatic impairment, or that her medications have affected those organs. Her fluid and electrolyte status is not questioned since none of her medications has major effects on that system. The same holds true for Mary's pulmonary, hematological, endocrine, gastrointestinal, neurological, dermatological, genitourinary, musculoskeletal, and psychological systems. Effects on her cardiac and eye, ear, nose, and throat systems are suspected, as evidenced by her hypotension and nasal congestion. Serzone and Afrin are possible causes.

Based on this evaluation, Mary's pharmacist has identified the following drug therapy problems in Mary:
- *Inappropriate compliance with Afrin Nasal Spray and Vancenase AQ. In each case, this is an actual drug therapy problem.*
- *Adverse effects from Afrin and Serzone causing nasal congestion and hypotension. The pharmacist believes these to be actual problems.*
- *Dosage too high with Benadryl. Although there is no direct evidence of a problem, the pharmacist believes that this dosage is potentially unsafe.*
- *Duration of therapy too long with Benadryl. Mary has been taking Benadryl as a sleep aid for several months. Again, there is no evidence of damage, so the pharmacist labels this a potential drug therapy problem.*

Chapter 5

◆

Patient Care Plan Development

A care plan is a course of action for helping a patient achieve a particular health-related goal. The care plan could be thought of as the "product" that the pharmaceutical care practitioner delivers: a concrete process for optimizing a patient's health and well-being.

To create a care plan, the pharmacist works with the patient—and other health care providers as appropriate—to identify, evaluate, and choose methods for ensuring that drug therapy is effective and for minimizing health-related problems. After completing a systematic evaluation of the patient, the pharmacist actively considers the patient's needs and determines "desirable outcomes" that both the pharmacist and patient agree on. The activities necessary to achieve these outcomes are then synthesized into a care plan, which the pharmacist documents in the patient's pharmacy record. When the situation warrants, the pharmacist reviews the plan and desirable outcomes with the patient's other health care providers.

Patients with multiple diseases or conditions may have care plans with various components addressing each condition. To make good decisions, the patient should be educated about the pros and cons of drug therapy options, such as cost, side effects, and monitoring-related factors. Of course, pharmacists should feel free to offer their professional judg-

> ## A New Way of Practicing
>
> Developing a care plan is absolutely vital if a pharmacist is to provide pharmaceutical care. Historically, although all pharmacists gathered at least some patient information, and found occasional drug therapy problems, they did not routinely develop a means by which to resolve problems. Instead, they would simply inform the physician of the problem and let the physician decide what should be done about it. In contrast, pharmaceutical care requires pharmacists to *accept responsibility for a patient's drug-related outcomes.*

ment about the options that are the most beneficial. Essential elements of the plan, including the patient's responsibilities in carrying it out, must be carefully and completely explained to increase the likelihood of compliance. Ultimately, the patient must agree with the care plan the pharmacist develops. If patients object to their care plans, for any reason, they are less likely to adhere and may have a poor outcome.

SETTING THERAPEUTIC GOALS

The first steps in developing a care plan are determining the outcome the pharmacist hopes to achieve—or, in other words, establishing a therapeutic goal—and then making sure the patient finds it acceptable. If the patient and pharmacist do not have similar goals, the patient is unlikely to comply with the care plan designed to achieve it.

Sometimes the goals a patient has in mind are unrealistic, which means the pharmacist must provide significant education to get the patient to realize the limits of what may be accomplished. Other times, the patient's goals are not unreasonable, but simply different from those of the pharmacist or physician. For example, a patient prescribed a cholesterol-lowering agent to be taken twice daily was taking only one tablet per day. On this therapy, he reduced his cholesterol from 430 mg/dl to 260 mg/dl. From the patient's perspective, this drop in cholesterol was sufficient to accomplish his goals for therapy, which were to lower his cholesterol as much as possible while only taking one tablet per day. The patient felt that his physician did not actually have a goal for therapy and was simply, as he stated it, "chasing numbers." Although the pharmacist tried

> ### PHARMACEUTICAL CARE GOALS MAY DIFFER FROM 'TRADITIONAL' GOALS
>
> Many pharmacists first learn about "goals" in therapeutics class, and some—especially clinically oriented practitioners—are accustomed to working with physicians to establish goals for therapy. Although the goals taught in therapeutics courses or set by clinical pharmacists often complement the goals of pharmaceutical care practitioners, they tend to be more narrowly focused and are usually related to an objective parameter, such as a laboratory assessment. Examples would be establishing a target hemoglobin A1c level for a patient with diabetes or setting a goal international normalized ratio for a patient on anticoagulant therapy. Although these are rational, defensible goals for therapy, most pharmacists do not participate in drug-use decision making at a level that involves them in setting such goals. Goals in pharmaceutical care are generally broader, which allows them to be set independent of the practice site.

to impress upon the patient that a further decrease in serum cholesterol was highly desirable, the patient remained unconvinced. Since his goals were being met, he had little interest in the goals of the pharmacist or physician.

The pharmacist must also consider the physician's goals for therapy. Unfortunately, these may not be readily apparent to the pharmacist or they may not be explicit. In such cases, the pharmacist will need to inform the physician of the pharmaceutical goals for therapy to ensure that the pharmacist and physician are not working at cross-purposes.

Even when the patient, pharmacist, and physician have mutual goals, they may phrase them completely differently, so the goals seem at first to be dissimilar. Pharmacists should look carefully for areas of common interest among goals. For example, a patient had poorly controlled diabetes and significant nocturia. The physician's goal was to decrease the patient's bedtime serum glucose level. The pharmacist wanted to improve the patient's quality of life. The patient simply claimed he wanted "to stop peeing at night." Although these goals all sound very different, they were readily reconciled so that each party achieved his goal by using a mutually agreeable care plan.

ILL-DEFINED GOALS

The first few times a pharmacist develops patient-specific goals, they tend to be vague. To avoid this trap, pharmacists must ensure that their goals are achievable, measurable, and consistent with their professional responsibilities. For example, after interviewing and evaluating a patient with poorly controlled hypertension, a pharmacist determines that the patient has a drug therapy problem of noncompliance with his medications. If the pharmacist is just beginning to provide pharmaceutical care, she may initially devise goals like "control patient's blood pressure" or "improve compliance." Although these seem reasonable, on further inspection it is apparent that there is no way to tell when such a goal has been accomplished. What does "control" mean? Suppose the patient improves his compliance from taking 50% of doses correctly to 60%. Does this change mean the goal has been met?

Goals must be well defined. Since the pharmacist has not explicitly defined her goals for the patient, there is no way to determine if they have been achieved—and thus they are not achievable. Blood pressures and compliance can be objectively evaluated and are measurable, but the target measures have not been stated.

An experienced pharmaceutical care practitioner would probably state the goals this way:

- "The patient demonstrates an understanding of the need for compliance with his drug therapy and refills 80% of his prescriptions within five days of the appropriate refill date."
- "Slow progression of hypertension complications by helping the patient take enough of his medication to maintain BP <140/90."

Such goals are achievable, since the pharmacist should readily be able to educate the patient about the risks of uncontrolled hypertension and the importance of compliance. They are measurable, since the refill target date is explicitly stated and easily evaluated, and blood pressure is easily monitored. They are also consistent with the responsibilities of the pharmaceutical care provider.

DEFINING GOALS

Pharmacists must ensure that their goals are:

- Achievable
- Measurable
- Consistent with their professional responsibilities.

The example above also demonstrates how to measure a goal for an outcome that is not really measurable. If a patient has gastric upset from a nonsteroidal antiinflammatory agent, there is no truly objective method to measure the pain relief resulting from the care plan. Therefore the measurement becomes either the patient's voiced complaints or his level of understanding. For the patient with hypertension, the phrase "the patient demonstrates" is as good a measure as can be defined. For the patient with gastric pain, a statement that "the patient no longer complains of stomach pain" defines the measurement. If a goal cannot be readily measured, it should focus on the patient's understanding of the situation, or the patient's subjective decrease in symptoms.

CONFUSING GOALS WITH METHODS

A common pitfall as pharmacists learn to set goals for therapy is to confuse the goal with its method of implementation; that is, incorrectly defining the care plan as the goal. For example, suppose a pharmacist evaluating a patient learns that red wine is a consistent trigger for her migraine headaches. The goal of therapy is not to educate the patient and convince her to stop drinking red wine. That is the plan. The goal is that the patient no longer complains of unacceptable numbers of migraine headaches. Although the distinction between goal and plan may seem obvious in retrospect, in practice pharmacists frequently confuse the two.

PRIORITIZING PROBLEMS

After the pharmacist has identified patient-specific goals that are achievable, measurable, professionally responsible, and not confused with the care plan itself, it is time to prioritize the goals according to their importance in the patient's care. The following criteria should be taken into consideration when setting priorities:

- Acuity of problems,
- Seriousness of problems,
- Patient's perceptions of seriousness and urgency of problems,
- The potential to correct problems,
- Appropriateness of the pharmacist's addressing this problem.

This step will not always be necessary because most patients will have only one drug therapy problem. In some patients, however, the pharmacist will find multiple problems.

When these criteria are used properly, one sees that the most serious problem does not necessarily have to be addressed first. Consider a patient with prostate cancer whose disease has not fully responded to chemotherapy and has metastasized to the bones. An oral narcotic is controlling his bone pain well but has led to constipation; the patient has not had a bowel movement in five days. Since his bone pain is currently well controlled, the pain does not represent a drug therapy problem at present. The patient's two drug therapy problems are:

> **SOLVE MULTIPLE PROBLEMS ONE AT A TIME**
>
> When patients have multiple drug therapy problems, pharmacists sometimes take on too much and try to solve them all at once. This almost always is not the best approach. In many cases, a patient will have suffered from the problems for a considerable period of time. Except when problems are both acute and serious, pharmacists usually have time to address them one by one. When pharmacists try to do too much at once, it is generally not clear which interventions resulted in which outcomes. Thus it can be hard to assess each outcome and determine if another intervention is needed. Usually pharmacists should address one or two problems at a time and come back to the remaining problems later.

- He needs additional therapy for his cancer.
- He suffers from the adverse effect of constipation caused by a narcotic.

The patient's most serious problem is the first one, since it has the most potential for a poor outcome—in this case, death. His most acute problem, however, is constipation. Because the clinical course of his cancer is likely to be much slower than the progression of complaints secondary to constipation, his bowel problems may be addressed before the cancer-related problems. The cancer is serious, but the constipation is more acute. No one ever died of constipation, but in the short term it is likely to have a greater negative impact on this patient's quality of life than his life-threatening cancer.

The last criterion on the list is also important in this case. Problems related to cancer or pain management may be beyond a particular pharmacist's level of competence and expertise. If so, it would be best for the pharmacist to focus on the patient's constipation since she may be the most appropriate health professional to resolve it—and may have greater interest than other health professionals in such a seemingly minor problem. Even if the pharmacist were skilled in managing cancer pain, should the bone pain become responsive only to radiation therapy, it is not correctable from the pharmacist's perspective because it is beyond the effects of drug therapy.

A key question to consider is whether a problem is correctable by a pharmacist using the tools a pharmacist has available. If the answer is no, then the problem is a low priority for the pharmacist. But this does not necessarily mean the problem is insignificant. A low-priority problem for the pharmacist may be a high-priority problem for the patient or physician. If it is, the pharmacist must refer the patient for medical care. Each health care professional should work on the problems for which he or she is best suited, with the common goal of resolving all the patient's drug therapy and medical problems.

OVERVIEW OF CARE PLANNING

Once pharmacists have developed a care plan, they have completed the third step in the Care Cycle. While creating the plan, the pharmacist integrates everything she knows about patients, their pathophysiology, the social or economic factors that relate to their health, the health care system, and drugs—including pharmacology, therapeutics, chemistry, and dosage forms. Care plan development requires that pharmacists consider all these features and use them to identify the best way to resolve the patient's drug therapy problems.

Initially, pharmacists should not censor themselves when designing a care plan. All possible interventions should be considered and then the best choice made. Pharmacists should ask themselves, "Given everything I know about this patient, the health care system, and drug therapy, what are all the possible things I could do?" Then they should ask, "Out of all these options, what is the best thing for me to do?"

When considering options, pharmacists should evaluate possible alternatives and work with patients and, when appropriate, other health care providers to choose the best course. Avoid rushing to accept the first solution that comes to mind, as there are usually at least two options for every drug therapy problem.

If drug therapy is to be modified, the pharmacist should investigate therapeutic alternatives in order to balance efficacy, safety, and cost. Taking the time to know the patient and develop a professional relationship will make it easier to weigh these factors. Cost or complexity of therapy may affect some patients' compliance, as may the psychosocial aspects of a disease or specific patient preferences.

POOR CARE PLANS

When pharmacists devise a poor care plan, it is typically because they have not taken the time to reflect on everything they know and examine their options. They latch on to the first seemingly reasonable method for resolving the patient's drug therapy problem, and this becomes the care plan. Keep in mind that the most obvious intervention may not be the best one. For example, in a patient with significant esophageal strictures who has extreme difficulty swallowing most solid dosage forms, the most obvious plan would be switching to a liquid dosage form. But because liquid dosage forms are often more expensive than equipotent doses of a tablet or capsule, this "obvious" care plan may not be the best one in a patient on a limited income and without prescription insurance. Another "obvious" care plan—having the patient crush the tablet and take it in jelly— would be equally irrational when dealing with a sustained release product that must not be crushed.

> **QUESTIONS TO ASK YOURSELF**
>
> • "Given everything I know about this patient, the health care system, and drug therapy, what are all the possible things I could do?"
>
> • "Out of all these options, what is the best thing for me to do?"

A care plan must start from the beginning by ensuring that the patient does, in fact, need the drug. If the answer is no, then the issue of dosage form is irrelevant. Pharmacists developing care plans must be sure they use all the information available to avoid settling for easy answers that may not be best for the patient.

ADDITIONAL RESEARCH

Sometimes additional research may be necessary to come to a decision about drug therapy options. Areas the pharmacist may need to research include:

- The patient's disease,
- Consequences to the patient of a particular drug therapy program,
- Usual drug and nondrug therapies,
- Dosages, adverse effects, and interactions of usual therapies.

After researching, the pharmacist should consider how the patient's unique combination of characteristics fits into the "big picture" of the disease state(s) and condition(s) the patient suffers from. Consider, for example, patients with cystitis. The pharmacist may need to review how the management of specific patients differs depending on individualized characteristics. Although the underlying pathophysiology, consequences of infection, and general antibiotic choices will be similar in most patients with cystitis, patients who are pregnant, on theophylline, or who have had multiple infections have special considerations that make their management unique. The choice of drug, dosage interval, or duration of therapy may differ for different patients, all of whom have the same infection. If the pharmacist is not aware of how patients' specific conditions may affect their care plans, it is necessary to research the possible options and choose the best one.

PATIENT-FOCUSED INTERVENTIONS

As pharmacists begin to gain expertise at developing care plans, they soon see that two basic types of interventions may be made: patient focused or drug focused.

Patient-focused interventions include assisting the patient with compliance problems, providing patient education, monitoring the patient, or implementing nondrug therapy such as a weight control program. Patient-focused interventions typically do not require the physician's permission to implement. Nevertheless, most pharmacists elect to keep physicians informed about patient-focused interventions and the drug therapy problems being targeted.

Depending on the pharmacist's particular practice, some patient-focused interventions may be quite in-depth and formalized. This may be especially true for pharmacists who offer disease management programs for asthma, weight loss, or other conditions. A well-designed disease management program will include specific educational or patient-monitoring interventions that the pharmacist will perform in a consistent, systematic fashion. In an asthma program, for example, the pharmacist may teach the patient about dust control, pets, asthma triggers, smoking cessation, peak flow monitoring, or inhaler technique—interventions that are entirely educational and not related to a drug. They would be presented as well-thought-out educational and monitoring plans with defined outcomes, not casual discussions that the pharmacist performs "off the cuff."

Educational interventions need not always be so complex. When assisting with compliance problems, for example, most pharmacists will not establish a formal compliance clinic. Instead, they will provide general education on the patient's drugs and diseases, discuss the need for compliance, and perhaps furnish compliance aids such as pill boxes or dosing calendars.

Patient-focused interventions may also involve referring a patient for medical care. Although pharmacists have performed this service for years, in a pharmaceutical care practice they are able to provide additional information to let the physician know how they evaluated the problem; what, if anything, has been done about it so far; and what recommendations the pharmacist has.

DRUG-FOCUSED INTERVENTIONS

Drug-focused interventions require some type of change in a patient's drug therapy. Potential changes are adding, discontinuing, or changing a drug, or changing a dose, dosage interval, or dosage form. Unless the drug-focused intervention involves a nonprescription medication, most will require the physician's cooperation to implement.

When a pharmacist intends to make a drug-related intervention, it is important to be specific. Recommendations that are too vague are not useful. For example, suggesting to a physician that a patient with early diabetes-related renal impairment be started on an angiotensin-converting enzyme inhibitor is not very helpful because it makes the physician responsible for choosing the drug, dose, dosage form, and duration of therapy. Pharmacists must make their suggestions as explicit as possible, even if it requires considerable time to research a disease and its treatment.

Besides being practically useless to the physician, making a nonspecific suggestion raises the possibility that the physician could choose a therapy that results in a new drug-related problem. For example, if the pharmacist simply suggested that the physician start the patient with early renal impairment on captopril, the physician might choose too low a dose.

It is in the area of drug-related interventions that pharmacists are particularly cautioned against making too many changes at once. Since drugs have such powerful and complex effects, the therapeutic response for one condition may result in an adverse effect on another condition. Ideally, pharmacists work with physicians to observe the response to one change in drug therapy before embarking on a second change. Some patients will be sufficiently ill that multiple drug-related interventions are indicated, but in most patients, one change at a time is usually the better plan.

'DO NOTHING' INTERVENTIONS

One final form of intervention is not really drug or patient focused. Known as the "do nothing" option, it is a bit of a misnomer. Historically, because pharmacists did not identify and resolve drug therapy problems in a consistent manner, "do nothing" was essentially a default action they unknowingly took as a result of not necessarily being aware that anything had to be done. In a pharmaceutical care practice, however, "do nothing" is a considered, deliberate decision resulting from the pharmacist's determination that no action is better than doing anything else. It is a form of patient monitoring similar to the "watchful waiting" described in Chapter 4. Although the "do nothing" option is rarely the correct choice for a patient, it should be considered and deliberately ruled out before proceeding to other interventions.

FINAL STEPS

One of the last steps in developing a care plan is formulating a strategy for measuring the success of the outcomes that have been set. This strategy should provide both objective and subjective information. Finally, the pharmacist should review the plan with the patient, indicating specifically what outcomes the patient should expect from drug therapy. It is very important for the pharmacist to speak at the appropriate level for the patient and make sure the patient understands how to incorporate the drug

---

PHARMACISTS' FEARS IN CARE PLANNING

Pharmacists often hesitate to devise and implement care plans until they feel they are pharmaceutical care experts. Presumably, this is because they lack confidence in their therapeutic knowledge base or patient management skills. Pharmacists who do not yet feel comfortable with pharmaceutical care may decide that action is not indicated, and that they will "monitor" the patient until the problem appears serious enough to require a more active intervention. This is a misuse of the term monitoring. The pharmacist is responding to a fear that action carries a potential for risk; that by doing something, the pharmacist could actually make things worse.

Although such fears are not unreasonable, most pharmacists never consider the reverse. Sometimes, not acting also carries a potential for risk. The literature suggests that a substantial number of hospital admissions are due to drugs, and that drug therapy problems cost the U.S. health care system billions of dollars a year. The pharmacist is well positioned to assist with these problems, but to do so, must act.

Pharmacists must remember that although pharmaceutical care draws on knowledge of drugs and diseases, the two are not synonymous. Pharmacists trained in pharmaceutical care have repeatedly demonstrated the ability to find and resolve drug therapy problems irrespective of their knowledge base, age, practice setting, or pharmacy degree. The more pharmacists know about drugs and diseases, the more problems they will find, and the more varied their solutions will be. Even so, all pharmacists have the basic tools to find and resolve at least some drug therapy problems. They all have the potential to do good things for patients. Fearful pharmacists are reminded of the maxim, "Do not let the perfect be the enemy of the good." If pharmacists wait until they are entirely comfortable with all aspects of care planning before intervening in patient care, the serious drug-related problems facing the health care system will not be resolved.

therapy into his or her everyday life. To ensure patient understanding, it is helpful to ask the patient to explain the process back to the pharmacist.

IMPLEMENTING CARE PLANS

When providing pharmaceutical care, it is essential to ensure that the patient has the means to comply with the pharmacist's care plan. In other words, the pharmacist must verify that the patient has the drugs, supplies, and information necessary to carry out the plan. If verification does not take place and the care plan is not properly implemented, the desired goals for therapy will not be achieved.

It should not be assumed that once the pharmacist has told the patient what to do, the patient will simply do it. If patients are left to gather supplies, contact the physician, and then go home to decide how to proceed, rarely will they be able to follow the pharmacist's care plan— and a poor outcome will generally result.

Implementing a care plan is a cooperative effort. The pharmacist must coordinate between the patient and physician to be certain that all parties understand what is required of them and that they know when various aspects of patient care and monitoring will occur.

PATIENT-FOCUSED CARE PLANS

Implementing a patient-focused care plan is not particularly complicated, especially if the pharmacist has established a therapeutic relationship with a patient who has consented to follow the plan. It only remains for the pharmacist to:

- Verify the patient's understanding of the plan.
- See that the patient has the necessary drugs and supplies.
- Make sure that the patient understands the need for follow-up.
- Make sure the patient will participate in monitoring.

On occasion, the pharmacist may perform these activities with one of the patient's family members or another caregiver if, for example, the patient is a child or is elderly and incapacitated. Since the physician is not typically involved to any great extent with a patient-focused care plan, the pharmacist usually needs only to inform the physician of what was done, not gain permission to proceed.

ENSURE UNDERSTANDING

When making sure that patients have a good understanding of their drug therapy, the pharmacist must verify that they know how to take their medications and then correct any misperceptions. Thinking back to the three Public Health Service questions in Chapter 3 is helpful (see page 32). During the patient interview, patients should have been able to explain to the pharmacist how much they understand—what the medications are for, exactly how to take them, and what to expect. If, during the patient interview, the pharmacist learns that a patient does not understand these basics, then correcting knowledge deficits becomes an initial step in implementing the care plan.

Tailoring explanations to the patient's level of comprehension is critical. In some cases, pharmacists may need to employ teaching aids, such as visual devices, graphics, or brochures, to supplement instruction. The best teaching technique is modeling; if possible, have the patient demonstrate the correct administration of the drug. To test patient understanding, the pharmacist should have the patient explain the information back and show the pharmacist how to administer the drug. Some patients may become irritated at being asked to repeat explanations, interpreting this request as a suggestion that the pharmacist thinks they did not understand the teaching. To avoid this problem, pharmacists may wish to preface their request by stating that this is done to be sure the pharmacist did not leave anything out.

> ### REPEATING FOR UNDERSTANDING
>
> To ensure understanding, patients should be asked to repeat instructions back to the pharmacist. A palatable way to make this request is, "To be sure I didn't leave out anything important, would you mind telling me [or showing me] how you will use your medication?"

Educating patients about their diseases may be handled in a similar way. Such education is especially important for patients with compliance problems related to misunderstandings about their medical condition. It is during disease state education that care plans related to lifestyle modifications are typically put into effect.

LIFESTYLE-RELATED PLANS

Lifestyle-related care plans are common since virtually everyone agrees on the wisdom of losing weight, stopping smoking, eating right, and getting more sleep and exercise. These are, however, among the most difficult interventions for pharmacists to implement and for patients to comply with. Patient-focused interventions that involve lifestyle changes require ongoing patient contact and reassurance. Formal disease management programs are attractive when lifestyle changes are part of the plan because they give both the pharmacist and patient a series of steps to follow. Informally encouraging patients to stop smoking or lose weight is rarely successful; most people already know they should make these changes. As with drug therapy education, the pharmacist should use whatever tools are helpful and then be sure that the patient demonstrates understanding.

MONITORING MECHANISMS

Working with the patient to develop and implement monitoring mechanisms helps ensure that the patient can and will comply with the necessary drug therapy or disease monitoring. If objective drug therapy monitoring tools such as laboratory testing, blood pressure monitoring, peak flow meters, or home glucose monitors will be employed, the pharmacist should see that arrangements for such monitoring have been made and are understood by the patient. This may include obtaining devices, explaining their use, and keeping records that the pharmacist or physician can evaluate with the patient during follow-up sessions. Again, demonstrating the equipment and having the patient explain back and show correct usage is an excellent way to determine if the patient will be able to carry out the monitoring plan.

> ### VERIFYING DRUGS, SUPPLIES
>
> Verifying that the patient has, or can obtain, all the necessary drugs, devices, and supplies necessary to follow the care plan is essential. This activity is especially important when patients will use a different source for these goods than the pharmacist who is providing pharmaceutical care. The pharmacist should also consider the patient's financial and insurance status to be certain they do not represent barriers to following a care plan.

COMPLEX CASES

For patients with more complicated diseases and therapies, pharmacists may have to implement a patient-focused care plan that includes several steps at the same time. For example, diabetic patients who require insulin and home blood glucose testing should be educated about:

- The effects of insulin on their disease state,
- Timing and amount of insulin injected,
- Correct injection technique,
- Correct storage of insulin,
- Overall expected results,
- Side effects of insulin,
- How to counteract a hypoglycemic reaction,
- Precautions necessary for diabetics on insulin.

The pharmacist should also make sure that patients possess the appropriate home blood glucose testing equipment and supplies and know how to use them, have the necessary medications and insulin syringes, and understand—and are willing and able to fulfill—their therapy plans.

FINAL CHECK

The last step is a final check to ensure that all the patient's follow-up activities are coordinated. The pharmacist must verify the following:

- Patients have set up any necessary follow-up appointments with their physicians.
- Patients know where and when to report for further laboratory monitoring.
- A date, time, and mechanism have been established for follow-up with the pharmacist.

DRUG-FOCUSED CARE PLANS

With the exception of care plans related to nonprescription medications, drug-focused care plans usually require the physician's cooperation. Consequently, they are more complex to implement. The first step is ensuring that the patient understands and has agreed to the drug-therapy changes that the pharmacist has proposed. Then the pharmacist can contact the physician to propose the changes. These suggestions must be as specific as possible. Pharmacists should outline their recommendations to physicians in the following areas:

- Drug,
- Dose,
- Dosage form,
- Duration of therapy,
- Appropriate monitoring parameters,
- Who will perform the monitoring and when.

PATIENTS DELIVERING CARE PLANS

There are several ways to contact the physician to implement a care plan. Often patients will insist that they see the physician themselves and discuss the pharmacist's care plan directly with the doctor. This scenario is most likely when there is no urgent or serious problem that needs immediate correction or when the patient has a scheduled physician appointment coming up soon. Pharmacists must be respectful of such patient preferences. Information from patient focus groups has shown that, although patients support the concept of pharmaceutical care and appreciate the pharmacist's actions, they clearly do not want the pharmacist to interfere with the physician-patient relationship.

When patients implement drug-focused care plans by communicating directly with their physicians, there is a risk that patients will deliver the pharmacist's message incorrectly, incompletely, or with the emphasis misplaced. Imagine the physician's response if the patient said, "The pharmacist told me to tell you to increase my dosage of metoprolol." To avoid such potential disasters, pharmacists should commit care plans to paper and have the patient take a copy to the physician's office. This allows patients to maintain autonomy while still giving pharmacists a degree of control over how their intentions are communicated to the physician.

PROPOSE SOLUTIONS TO DEVELOP PROFESSIONAL RELATIONSHIPS WITH PHYSICIANS

For pharmacists to work cooperatively with physicians, a mutually respectful professional relationship is necessary. Unfortunately, some pharmacist-physician relationships lack this quality. A key reason? The most common contact physicians have with pharmacists—outside of prescription refill requests—is when pharmacists call to inform them of patient allergies, previous adverse effects, conflicts with third party formularies, or patients who cannot afford a drug. In each case, the pharmacist is *informing the physician of a problem.* The potential unspoken message is that the physician erred in prescribing, or else this problem would not have happened. Pharmacists do not intend to convey this message but it is largely unavoidable. If every phone call pharmacists received from physicians pointed out dispensing problems, pharmacists would not want to talk to physicians very much, either.

When pharmacists call to point out a problem, they rarely describe it succinctly, outline why it is important to both the patient and the physician, and then recommend a resolution that is based on patient-specific knowledge. Instead, pharmacists typically let physicians know there is a problem and then fall silent. To the unspoken message, "You made a mistake," the pharmacist

adds, "And what do you propose to do about it?"

Although pharmaceutical care practice still requires that pharmacists inform physicians of drug therapy problems, smart practitioners try to change the dynamics of the relationship.

- They meet with local physicians to inform them of changes they are making in their practices to better assist their mutual patients.

- They explain how pharmacists can help physicians by taking over some of the time-consuming educational activities that busy physicians may not have time for.

- They consistently demonstrate that they are making these changes to *help patients.*

Even practitioners who are not able to actively market themselves to the local medical community can take a vital step to change the pharmacist-physician relationship: *Whenever they contact a physician to discuss a drug therapy problem, they propose a solution.* Once physicians understand that pharmacists are interested in and capable of solving problems, rather than just pointing them out, a relationship between professional colleagues is likely to ensue.

DISCUSSING PLANS BY PHONE

Most drug-focused care plans are implemented after the pharmacist has discussed the plan with the physician by telephone. This approach requires pharmacists to clearly organize the message they wish to send and how they want to send it. When contacting physicians by telephone, it is imperative that pharmacists:

- Know what they want to say before making the call.
- Have at least one solution for every drug therapy problem discussed.
- Consider ahead of time how the call may sound to a physician who is unaware that a problem exists.

Many pharmacists who try to telephone physicians express considerable frustration at not being able to navigate through the various layers of personnel in the medical office. They wonder if staff members actively try to prevent them from speaking with the physician. Make no mistake: slowing down access to the physician is a large part of their job. A physician's time is both scarce and expensive. There has to be a convincing reason to let the pharmacist through all the barriers, and too often, the pharmacist does not provide one. Pharmacists who get through typically have developed a solid relationship with the physician and have demonstrated that it is worth the physician's time to accept their phone calls.

Some pharmacists get through by using drug-related jargon beyond the comprehension of receptionists and even some nurses. If office staff do not understand what the pharmacist is talking about but believe it to be serious, they may forward the call directly to the physician. This approach is not for the fainthearted or the beginner; pharmacists who use it must be absolutely certain of what they are talking about. And they should be sure the problem is important. If it isn't, this method will not work again.

CONVEYING PLANS IN WRITING

A good method for sharing the care plan is to contact the physician in writing, either by fax or by mail. This method has many advantages:

- It allows pharmacists to think through the care plan thoroughly, because it must be written down. They can consider exactly what they want to tell the physician and the best way to say it.
- The physician can contemplate the pharmacist's suggestions at length without having to react immediately in response to a telephone call.
- The letter serves as a form of documentation that the pharmacist and physician can keep in the patient's chart as a record of their activities.

COMMUNICATION TIP: KNOW WHAT YOU WANT TO SAY

Developing drug-focused care plans is sometimes easier than employing the communication skills necessary to implement them. Too often, pharmacists phone the physician's office before they have worked out everything they want to say. Even when they have established a defensible care plan, they may neglect to "sell" it to the physician appropriately.

For example, when interviewing a patient, a pharmacist learned that she had diabetic gastroparesis that was being treated with cisapride. Although cisapride worked well and was not causing any problems, the patient was on a fixed income and, in an attempt to save money, only took her cisapride when her symptoms were severe. Consequently, her disease was not being well controlled and she frequently had stomach pain.

The pharmacist's care plan called for the cisapride to be changed to metoclopramide and he contacted the physician to ask for the medication to be changed. The physician refused. The pharmacist was surprised; he had identified a serious problem and developed a good care plan. Why wouldn't the physician cooperate?

The physician's perspective was this: He had received a phone call from a pharmacist he did not know, about a patient he had not seen in several months, asking to change a medication that he was not aware was causing problems. This attempt to implement a care plan had no context—it was simply a phone call from out of the blue.

Had the physician clearly understood that the patient's disease was poorly controlled because she could not afford her medicine, which therefore was not achieving the intended therapeutic effect, it would have made a big difference. Any reasonable physician recognizes that a poor outcome needs to be corrected. But the pharmacist did not outline the problem clearly, explain that he was using patient-specific knowledge, or emphasize that the problem was discovered by talking with the patient. If he had, the pharmacist's suggestion to change to a specific dosage of metoclopramide, and his offer to follow up with the patient to ensure that no further problems developed, would have been more warmly received.

If the pharmacist is not an experienced writer, it may take several drafts before an acceptable letter is produced. The pharmacist should be sure that the wording is clear and concise, yet thorough; that the problem is clearly stated; that a solution is proposed; and that nothing in the letter may inadvertently give offense. Because words on a page do not communicate a person's emotions and tone as well as the voice does, they run the risk of appearing disapproving or scolding. A poor choice of written words may offend someone even when the same words delivered orally do not cause problems. For wording suggestions, see the sample letter at the end of this chapter.

Keep in mind that although written communication is efficient and avoids some potential pitfalls of telephone interventions, it is slower than other options and is not recommended for urgent problems that require immediate attention.

ORGANIZING FOLLOW-UP MONITORING

The final step in the Care Cycle is following up with the patient to monitor the outcome of the care plan. To ensure that specific goals are met, the pharmacist will need to regularly monitor the patient's progress according to the strategy outlined in the patient's drug therapy plan. At predetermined intervals the pharmacist will review subjective and objective monitoring parameters to determine if satisfactory progress is being made and if further drug therapy problems have developed. Patient monitoring is similar in some ways to the data gathering carried out during the initial pharmaceutical care visit, but is more focused.

If the desired outcomes are not being met, or if new problems have occurred, the pharmacist, physician, and patient may need to discuss possible changes in the drug therapy plan. Changes may be warranted to maintain or enhance the safety or effectiveness of drug therapy, or to minimize overall health care costs.

WHEN TO FOLLOW UP

First, the pharmacist should determine exactly when to follow up on a patient's progress. Criteria to consider include:

- Expected time course before a therapeutic effect is seen,
- Expected time course before an adverse effect is seen,
- Time to onset of a possible drug interaction,
- Natural course of the disease,
- Length of time drug therapy will be required,
- Likelihood of additional drug therapy problems and their importance.

In establishing times to follow up with patients, the type of disease state and the specific patient's risk factors should be weighted heavily. For instance, patients taking medication for acute conditions may be contacted within a few hours or after several days, depending on the length and purpose of the drug therapy. However, patients taking medications for chronic conditions usually need to be contacted several times:

1. Five to ten days after beginning therapy,

2. One month after initial follow-up,

3. Every three to six months during ongoing therapy.

Patients at a high risk of drug therapy problems may need more frequent follow-up visits.

COORDINATING WITH THE PATIENT

Next, the pharmacist needs to coordinate with the patient to establish a follow-up schedule and method. Because patients are not accustomed to having pharmacists monitor their clinical progress, it is important to inform them that a follow-up session is necessary. Patients who receive a phone call from the pharmacist without expecting one will tend to assume that there is a problem with their prescription. Or, if they are unaware that the pharmacist plans to call them and a third party answers, they may resent the loss of confidentiality. Patients have to know when the pharmacist will contact them and how.

FOLLOW-UP APPROACHES

The two basic approaches for patient follow-up are telephone calls and repeat visits to the pharmacy. When phone calls are to be used, the pharmacist must ensure that the patient's record includes the appropriate telephone number (home or workplace) and the best time to call. If the patient has particular concerns about confidentiality—as in the case of a teenage girl taking oral contraceptives—the record should also note whether it is acceptable to indicate to a third party that the pharmacist has called or whether it is permissible to leave a message with a family member or coworker.

If follow-up will be performed during a repeat visit to the pharmacy, it is best to use scheduled

> ### COMMUNICATION TIP: USE THE RIGHT WORDS
>
> Good communication is key to implementing drug-focused care plans. Pharmacists should be assertive but not aggressive. To avoid sparking defensiveness in the prescriber when making therapy suggestions, do not use the words "you" or "your," which imply blame and ill will. Focus on the patient, who is the common interest of both the physician and pharmacist. For instance, instead of saying, "The inhaler you prescribed is not working," say, "I'm concerned that the patient's breathing problems may require additional therapy."
>
> If, despite the pharmacist's best efforts, the prescriber refuses to change therapy, be polite. Avoid escalating the conversation into an exchange of who is "right" or "wrong." Keep the communication channels open so as not to inhibit interactions with the prescriber in the future. Explain the situation to the patient in a way that does not undermine the physician-patient relationship. Remember that reasonable people can disagree about pharmacotherapeutic choices.

appointments. This ensures that the pharmacist knows the patient is coming in and has set aside time to perform the follow-up. The disadvantage to follow-up appointments is that patients often forget to keep them. It may be a good idea to call patients the day before an appointment to remind them; keep in mind, however, that telephone reminders carry the same confidentiality risk as mentioned above.

Many pharmacists are initially concerned that they will need to do a follow-up evaluation each time the patient comes to the pharmacy for a prescription refill. Because most monitoring occurs at scheduled times, this concern is unwarranted. If a patient comes into the pharmacy between follow-up visits, the pharmacist should simply inquire briefly into the patient's progress by asking one or two open-ended questions, such as, "How has your drug therapy been working for you?" and "What new problems or concerns can I help you with?" If the medications seem to be working and the patient does not voice any new complaints, then the complete follow-up assessment can be performed at the scheduled time. If the patient indicates that there is a new drug therapy problem, the pharmacist can either address it immediately or move up the scheduled follow-up appointment.

After patients have been receiving pharmaceutical care for a while, they may be followed by the pharmacist for several concurrent drug therapy problems. It is highly advisable to coordinate all follow-ups so that the pharmacist and patient do not need to schedule repeated sessions. Delaying some follow-ups for a few days or weeks will help prevent patients from losing interest in pharmaceutical care because of too many repeat visits close together.

QUESTIONS TO CONSIDER DURING MONITORING

- *Drug effectiveness.* What are the signs that this drug is working effectively?
- *Adverse effects.* What are the signs of this drug's adverse effects?
- *Drug interactions.* What is the symptomatology of this drug's interactions with other drugs?
- *Compliance.* What are the signs and symptoms of noncompliance with therapy?

TRACKING CALLS AND APPOINTMENTS

Pharmacists must have a mechanism for tracking which follow-ups need to be performed on a given day. The mechanism will depend on the pharmaceutical workload unique to each practice. At first, a simple wall or desk calendar may be used to write down the names and phone numbers of patients to contact. The first thing each morning, the pharmacist can check her schedule and prepare for the day's activities. The day before, the pharmacy technician should pull the files of all patients who will be seen tomorrow and refile the updated files of patients who were seen yesterday.

In busier practices pharmacists are likely to use computer programs for documenting care, some of which have built-in calendar functions that set follow-up dates for patients and provide a written schedule of each day's follow-up activities. The technician can print out the appropriate information before a patient's visit, or the pharmacist can review the information on screen.

No matter how pharmacists follow up with patients, they should briefly review each patient's record before meeting with or telephoning the patient. Once they have more than a few pharmaceutical care patients in their practice, pharmacists often start to forget a patient's individual details. If patients get the impression that the pharmacist does not know the particulars of their case, it impairs the therapeutic relationship.

INFORMATION TO GATHER DURING FOLLOW-UP

Information the pharmacist needs to assess the effectiveness of therapy during a follow-up visit includes:

- Therapeutic efficacy of drug therapy,
- Safety of drug therapy,
- Drug interactions,
- Patient compliance,
- New problems of the patient,
- Unmet needs of the patient.

Answers to the questions in the box on page 96 will provide evidence of how well the care plan is working to achieve the therapeutic goals set earlier. They will also indicate if the drug therapy is causing any symptomatic adverse effects or drug interactions or if the patient has not complied with the care plan. As in the original data-gathering session described in Chapter 3, the pharmacist will collect both subjective and objective data and evaluate it. Once again, the pharmacist should start with open-ended questions and then narrow the scope with closed-ended questions. Unlike the pharmacist's initial interview with the patient, however, the questioning will focus more on drugs and diseases covered by the care plan.

If the pharmacist determines that the patient has not made clinical progress or that new drug therapy problems have arisen, she must work with the patient and physician to determine whether the original plan should be continued or modified. Some steps of the pharmaceutical care process may need to be repeated to help the patient work towards goals.

Continuing with the original care plan may be a good choice when there are compliance issues or when additional time may result in improvements. If the care plan is not working or if adverse effects or drug interactions have occurred, however, therapy may need to be modified.

If the initial interview showed that the patient's other diseases and drugs cause no problems, the follow-up visit need only confirm that no new problems have arisen with those diseases and drugs.

Only limited new data have to be collected during a follow-up session. The pharmacist should determine if patients have developed new medical conditions or have had changes in their drug therapy since the last visit. If they have, a focused interview should be performed to determine if the new diseases or changes in drug therapy have caused new drug therapy problems. Each time a new drug therapy problem is discovered, the Care Cycle begins again.

PROGRESS TOWARD GOALS

Monitoring the patient's progress toward therapeutic goals involves comparing patient information with objective and subjective monitoring parameters. The patient's progress should be documented in the chart. When goals are being met, the pharmacist should give the patient positive reinforcement. This may take the form of cheerful encouragement or pointing out and congratulating a patient on marked improvement, for example.

CASE STUDY

The pharmacist's job now is to develop and implement care plans for each of Mary Blythe's drug therapy problems. These problems are:

1. *Inappropriate compliance with Afrin Nasal Spray and Vancenase AQ.*
2. *Adverse effects from Afrin and Serzone, resulting in nasal congestion and hypotension.*
3. *Dosage too high with Benadryl.*
4. *Duration of therapy too long with Benadryl.*

The first thing the pharmacist must do is establish an achievable, measurable, and professionally responsible goal for each problem. At this point, these goals are not necessarily written down, but the pharmacist and others should be able to deduce the goals when reviewing documentation of the care session (see Chapter 6). Mary's pharmacist, working with her, devises the following three goals for therapy:

- *Mary will not have complaints regarding the signs and symptoms of allergies and nasal congestion.*
- *Mary will have relief of her depressive symptoms without acquiring new, bothersome adverse drug effects.*
- *Mary's symptoms of insomnia will be controlled to her satisfaction with minimal additional medications.*

Now that both Mary and the pharmacist agree on goals for therapy, they work together to prioritize Mary's problems. Although not particularly serious or urgent, her problems with compliance and adverse effects are of genuine concern

---

CASE STUDY

and thus are actual *problems as defined in Chapter 2. The dosage and duration of Benadryl therapy are considered* potential *problems, since currently there is no evidence of harm. Mary also is quite anxious to improve her nasal congestion. Therefore, she and the pharmacist elect to develop a plan today that will result in appropriate compliance with Afrin and Vancenase AQ and reduce the nasal congestion caused by Afrin and Serzone. Although Mary's blood pressure is worrisome, her depression has responded well to Serzone and she would like to stay on it if possible. The pharmacist concurs, but suggests to Mary that they inform her physician of the pharmacist's findings. Mary agrees to this approach.*

As for Mary's problems with Benadryl, she asks the pharmacist to develop a care plan that will be implemented only after she sees how well her congestion responds to changes in the Afrin and Vancenase AQ. Since the problems with Benadryl are potential, the pharmacist finds this acceptable.

How to Achieve Goals

The pharmacist must now decide how best to achieve the goals that have been set. The first thing he does is rule out the "do nothing" option. Mary's problems are causing her significant trouble breathing and there is good reason to believe that the benefits of an active intervention outweigh the risks. The pharmacist then considers various ways the therapeutic goals could be achieved.

In the case of inappropriate compliance and adverse effects caused by Afrin, the pharmacist could simply recommend that Mary stop taking Afrin. Given the current state of her breathing, and the slow onset of Vancenase AQ, however, Mary would likely have several days of unacceptable symptoms and eventually stop complying with the care plan. The pharmacist could recommend an oral decongestant such as pseudoephedrine. This, however, would result in the expense of additional drug therapy and could interfere with proper evaluation of Mary's possible blood pressure problems. Instead, the pharmacist decides that slowly tapering Mary off Afrin Spray is the best approach. He will suggest that, for the first week, Mary use her Afrin no more than twice daily and alternate nostrils for each dose. The second week, Mary will continue to alternate nostrils, but use the Afrin only once daily. By the third week, the Vancenase AQ should be fully effective and Mary should not need Afrin at all. If she still has congestion, she will use Afrin only once a day in one nostril and not for more than three days. If this is ineffective, the pharmacist will refer Mary to her physician for a medical evaluation.

CASE STUDY

As for Mary's poor compliance with Vancenase AQ, the pharmacist also considers several options. Changing to another nasal steroid or cromolyn is not indicated because, given the compliance problem, it is impossible to tell if Vancenase AQ has been effective. Recommending an oral steroid would be excessively risky at this time. Therefore, the pharmacist elects to develop a dosing reminder calendar for Mary and to educate her on the proper use of her nasal inhaler.

Since Mary prefers to continue on her Serzone for now, the pharmacist feels that the best approach is to write Mary's physician to relate what the pharmacist has learned. The alternative of not writing the prescriber is ruled out since the pharmacist feels that Mary's blood pressure is potentially serious enough to warrant medical intervention and, further, the pharmacist wishes to maintain a positive, collegial relationship with the physician.

Although Mary does not wish to change her Benadryl use at this time, the pharmacist elects to devise a care plan that can be implemented when Mary is more open to further changes. Several options are considered. Simply discontinuing Benadryl is ruled out since Mary has been on it for several consecutive months; it is also helping to control her allergies and aiding her sleep. Changing to another agent, such as doxylamine, offers no apparent advantage over Benadryl. Therefore, the pharmacist decides to gradually taper Mary's Benadryl 25 mg at a time at weekly intervals. Once Mary has been tapered off Benadryl, she is not to take more than 50 mg at bedtime when her allergies are troublesome. As for her insomnia, the pharmacist will educate Mary on sleep hygiene and supply her with a set of relaxation tapes that she can listen to in bed to help her fall asleep.

IMPLEMENTATION

Having developed a care plan for each problem, the pharmacist must now implement them. The care plans related to Afrin, Vancenase AQ, and Benadryl are all patient-focused interventions. Accordingly, the pharmacist needs only to educate Mary with the necessary information and does not need to contact the physician before proceeding. The pharmacist informs Mary about how nasal decongestants can actually make nasal congestion worse. The pharmacist outlines the Afrin tapering schedule that has been developed, including alternating nostrils, and makes sure that Mary agrees to it. Next, the pharmacist asks Mary to demonstrate her understanding of appropriate Afrin use by repeating the care plan back to him, which she is able to do.

CASE STUDY

For the Vancenase AQ, the pharmacist demonstrates appropriate use of the inhaler and asks Mary to demonstrate it as well. He then provides education about how nasal steroids prevent rather than treat allergic symptoms and explains why regular use is important. Mary appears to understand why proper compliance is important and agrees to follow the schedule outlined on the dosage calendar and to check off each time she uses it. Although the pharmacist knows that Mary will not presently make any changes in her Benadryl use, he briefly describes his suggestions, which she agrees to take under advisement. In the meantime, the pharmacist teaches Mary about good sleep hygiene and she agrees to purchase the relaxation tapes the pharmacist recommends.

Finally, the pharmacist informs Mary about the importance of a follow-up session to monitor her outcome. They agree that the pharmacist will telephone Mary at home in one week, since proper compliance with Vancenase AQ should give her some relief after a week's consistent use. At that time, the pharmacist will inquire about the clinical response of Mary's congestion, how much Afrin she is using, and her compliance with Vancenase AQ. The pharmacist will also evaluate whether increased use of Vancenase AQ is causing any problems, such as nasal dryness. The pharmacist will then inquire into Mary's Benadryl use to see if she is now willing to consider a dosage change, and will assess whether the relaxation tapes are helping with her sleep. Finally, the pharmacist will look into Mary's blood pressure issues. If she is still complaining of symptoms consistent with hypotension, the pharmacist will ask Mary to return to the pharmacy for a blood pressure check. Depending on the results, he may then refer Mary to her physician. As time goes on, the pharmacist will also verify that Mary's compliance with Vancenase AQ is meeting the target goal for compliance and that her use of Afrin is acceptable.

INFORMING THE PHYSICIAN

The last task is for the pharmacist to inform the physician about Mary's possible adverse effect with Serzone. Since the pharmacist is already writing a letter about Serzone, he elects to keep the physician informed about Mary's total pharmaceutical care plans. The letter he writes appears on page 102.

CASE STUDY

Concerned Physician, M.D.
Hospital Street
Home Town, USA

Dear Doctor:

I am writing to you about our patient, Mary Blythe. Mary came into
the pharmacy today for a refill of her Serzone prescription and also
complained of significant difficulty breathing, which she felt was caused
by her numerous allergies. After a brief interview with Mary I learned
that she suffers from depression, which she finds is well managed on her
Serzone 150 mg po BID. Mary has numerous environmental allergies for
which she has been prescribed Vancenase AQ. She also self-medicates her
allergies with Benadryl 100 mg po qhs and Afrin Spray, two sprays in each
nostril twice daily. She finds the Benadryl helpful for her insomnia as
well. Having evaluated Mary's drug therapy, I would like to inform you
about the following concerns.

Mary's nasal congestion may be largely due to her overuse of Afrin,
coupled with poor compliance with her Vancenase AQ. I have given
Mary a schedule to taper her Afrin use and have educated her on the
proper use of Vancenase AQ. Mary has agreed to limit her use of
decongestants and to improve her use of Vancenase AQ. I have provided
Mary with a schedule to decrease her Benadryl use. She is unwilling to do
so at this time, but will consider this in the future. Meanwhile, she will
use some relaxation tapes to help her sleep.

Finally, I noted that Mary had a blood pressure of 90/60 in the pharmacy
today. She also complains of occasional dizziness. As you know, Serzone
has alpha-adrenergic blocking properties. I am concerned that Serzone
may be affecting Mary's blood pressure as well as causing some nasal
congestion secondary to its alpha blocking effects. She has indicated that
she would prefer to stay on the Serzone for now. I will be checking with
Mary in one week to determine how well her allergies and sleeping habits
have responded to these suggestions. If she still complains of dizziness,
I will have her come into the pharmacy and check her blood pressure.
If it remains low, I will refer her to your office for medical assessment.

I trust that you will find this information useful. Please feel free to contact
me at 555-5678 if there is any more information that I can provide.

Sincerely,

A. Pharmacist, R.Ph.

Chapter 6

◆

Documentation

Documenting the patient care provided during a pharmaceutical care encounter is a critical step in the pharmaceutical care process. The act of documentation is an opportunity to contemplate and re-evaluate the data collected and the care plan generated for the patient. It also creates a valuable record for use in providing future care to the patient. No pharmacist is capable of remembering all the details regarding specific patients' care—details must be written down. Good records are also useful for audits conducted by third party payers and as legal evidence, should information about a patient's care ever be needed by the courts.

Documentation is a separate function from those discussed in the previous three chapters, occurring after data collection and evaluation, drug therapy problem-solving, and care plan development. Next to taking on new patient care responsibilities—which is an extension of what pharmacists already do—generating and maintaining a patient documentation system is the hardest task for pharmacists making the transition to pharmaceutical care. Like many other pharmaceutical care functions, creating useful and concise documentation requires a restructuring of the pharmacist's thought process.

MORE THAN COMPLETING FORMS

Documentation is much more than filling out forms as one interviews the patient. Data collection forms are helpful tools, but no "ideal" form is available for all patients and all situations. As mentioned in Chapter 3, pharmacists must guard against concentrating more on the form than on the patient during the patient encounter. Instead, they should take only enough notes to be able to reconstruct the patient encounter later. An exception would be when the pharmacist is entering detailed data directly onto a flow sheet that is a permanent part of the patient record.

Blood pressure and pulse rate are good examples of information that should be written down immediately to maintain accuracy. For efficiency, these can be noted directly in the patient's record.

Each patient's entire record, as well as pertinent information and comments regarding a patient's therapy, should be readily retrievable, or else the records will not be useful. Other caregivers in the pharmacy or institution must be able to understand and use the records with no trouble. Documenting events, such as how many drug interactions were caught in a day, or documenting isolated interventions, are not the same as creating usable patient records. In records that facilitate patient care, the following are quickly and easily found:

- An accurate history of the patient,
- A current care plan,
- Instructions about what should take place during the next patient encounter.

TYPES OF DOCUMENTATION SYSTEMS

Basic components of a patient record were outlined in the Omnibus Budget Reconciliation Act of 1990 (OBRA'90), a law that requires not only medication counseling for Medicaid patients but also the creation of records containing patient demographic information, a medication list, a listing of conditions or disease states, and comments on the patient's drug therapy. Although this type of record has been mandated since January 1993, the record-keeping systems in many pharmacies are not conducive to creating readily retrievable patient-specific information. Some pharmacists record comments on the back of the prescription order, which is a problem because its size limits the amount of information it can carry—and often it is filed away, never to be viewed again.

'If we didn't document it, we didn't do it—or at least we can't prove it' is a common sentiment among pharmaceutical care practitioners.

Although pharmacists often keep computer records, those allowed by dispensing systems—while steadily improving—tend to be inadequate for generating adequate patient care documentation. The record-keeping portions of dispensing software, where demographic information, medications, and medical conditions are listed, have the potential to be useful, but many do not allow sufficient space for comments on the patient's drug therapy. Cryptic notes created to fit in tiny data fields, which do not transmit complete thoughts, risk being more dangerous than helpful in caring for patients.

Today, several computer dispensing programs include pharmaceutical care modules that provide an improved format for documenting patient care. Some others link their programs to available pharmaceutical care documentation programs. Free-standing pharmaceutical care documentation programs are also available. Pharmacists should postpone decisions about buying a computerized documentation system until they have adequate experience in providing care and completing basic documentation. Which product or add-on is appropriate depends on the methods being used in providing patient care and the needs for documentation beyond what the pharmacist's current dispensing system offers. Issues to be considered in evaluating a documentation package are listed in the box below.

As pharmacists begin to provide pharmaceutical care, they discover not only that they need an efficient documentation system but also how challenging it is to create one. In many community pharmacies, the only documentation being done is signing the paperwork for controlled substances dispensed each day or recording information for transferred

---

ATTRIBUTES TO CONSIDER IN DOCUMENTATION PROGRAMS

Pharmacists would be wise to put off investing in computerized documentation software until they have enough pharmaceutical care experience to know what they really need. Because the market is in flux and published information quickly becomes outdated, the best way to identify vendors is to contact the American Society for Automation in Pharmacy, 492 Norristown Rd., Suite 160, Bluebell, PA 19422. Telephone: (610) 825-7686. When looking for a computer documentation software package, consider these issues:

- Overall ease of use,

- Complexity of entry,

- Time required to learn the system,

- Speed of entry,

- Usefulness for collecting and documenting relevant information,

- Ease with which documentation tasks can be delegated to clerical staff,

- Quality of report generation,

- Billing capabilities,

- Hardware requirements,

- The system's flexibility and ability to be customized,

- Ease of integration with current software,

- Vendor responsiveness to user needs,

- Technical support required from the vendor to set up the system, as well as to customize or upgrade it,

- Actual support provided,

- Cost,

- How often the system must be upgraded,

- Cost of upgrades,

- Network and multi-user capability.

prescriptions. Pharmacists are probably the only health care professionals who do not generate some kind of clinical record each time they provide care to a patient.

We recommend that pharmacists begin providing care with a simple paper documentation system and then investigate more expensive systems after they have a better sense of what will work for them. We jokingly say that pharmaceutical care can be provided using only a Big Chief writing tablet and a crayon.

How sophisticated the initial paper system should be depends on how long it will be used. If the system will be temporary, inexpensive manila folders work well. If the system is likely to become a permanent part of patient care it may be worth investing in one like those in other professional practices, which code charts by color, letter, and date. In either type of paper system there must be a way to affix pages in the chart so that patient data are not lost or disorganized. Right now, most pharmacies keep a "hard" or paper copy in addition to an electronic copy of patient records, but as time goes on and comfort level increases, this may change.

THE VALUE OF DOCUMENTATION

- Provides a permanent record of patient information that the pharmacist has collected and analyzed, as well as of the patient's care plan;

- Efficiently communicates key information to colleagues at the practice site and to other health care providers;

- Contributes to a repository of accumulated patient data;

- Provides evidence of the pharmacist's actions and successes in patient care;

- Serves as a legal record of care provided;

- Provides back-up for billing requests and furnishes answers to questions from third party payers.

PROBLEM-ORIENTED RECORDS

Experience gained from the medical community suggests that problem-oriented records are the most efficient and useful type. Developed in the early 1960s by Lawrence Weed,[1,2] the problem-oriented approach to documentation streamlines the amount of reading that practitioners must do to update themselves on a problem's status. The patient's medical chart is organized by medical problem and contains structured notes about each problem. Providers can determine the current diagnostic, therapeutic, and monitoring plans at a glance rather than having to extract them out of unformatted "stories" about the patient and the care provided.

In pharmacy practices, organizing charts by drug therapy problem is very effective. By writing structured notes about each drug therapy problem or closely related group of problems, pharmacists can quickly locate the most recent entry and read the portion devoted to the current plan and follow-up schedule. This speeds the process of deciding what to

---

GUIDELINES FOR PATIENT CHARTS

- The pharmacy record should include all the important demographic and historical information about the patient, as well as details about ongoing care. Some specifics to include:
  — address,
  — phone number,
  — birth date,
  — insurance information (including policy numbers),
  — other billing information.

- All sheets of paper should be identified by patient name or identification number in case they become separated from the chart. Information entered into a permanent patient record should never be removed.

- It is best to maintain one complete record for each patient, to be used for all care delivered to that patient. Generating separate records for different purposes is not only redundant and time consuming, but also tremendously inefficient because it means that multiple records must be consulted to find necessary information. Having only one record for each patient is not always achievable, but is a worthwhile goal.

- The record should be updated each time the pharmacist interacts with the patient, or whenever the pharmacist acquires additional information on the patient.

- Use caution when using abbreviations or other documentation shortcuts that could be misinterpreted by

other readers. Standard medical abbreviations are listed in a number of reference books, including *Medical Abbreviations: 12,000 Conveniences at the Expense of Communications and Safety*, 8th edition, by Neil M. Davis.

- Some pharmacists dictate their notes for patient records into a tape recorder for transcription by an assistant. When errors are found during review of transcribed or handwritten notes, or if changes are made for any reason, the original text should be retained in readable form; it should not be blacked or opaqued out. A good method is to put a single line through the error, write in the correction, and initial it. If simple editing is insufficient to correct errors in the chart, an addendum should be used for clarification. Once the note is signed by the care provider who generated it, no changes should be made to the note.

- Records created for patients should never be destroyed. If patients become "inactive"—that is, stop using the pharmacy for any reason—their charts may be removed from the active files and archived (microfiche is a space-saving option). Pharmacists can find out the requirements in their state for maintaining records and the statute of limitations for lawsuits by checking with their liability insurance provider or the state board of pharmacy.

do next and when to do it. If pharmacists need additional information to determine if the care plan is correct, they can review other relevant sections of the record to find material that justifies the assessment and plan. Eliminating extraneous material and "short stories" about patients speeds both documentation and interpretation of information.

PROBLEM-ORIENTED PHARMACY RECORDS

A problem-oriented pharmacy record (POPR) should conform to the guidelines in the box on page 107. It also should contain a problem list that briefly delineates the important information in the chart and serves as an index. As shown in the sample on page 109, called the Pharmaceutical Care Data Sheet, the form lists the patient's medical problems, medication allergies, current medications, and drug therapy problems.

The section on drug therapy problems should identify the type of problem and provide sufficient detail about the medication and problem encountered to clarify the situation (i.e., undesirable effect—nausea from aspirin). There should be a short explanatory note corresponding to each drug therapy problem.

The medical problem list should, as much as possible, convey medical diagnoses rather than symptoms.

A SAMPLING OF PAPER CHART SUPPLIERS

Here is a short list of vendors that supply paper charting systems. Pharmacists can also contact physicians' offices or clinics to identify potential suppliers.

BIBBERO SYSTEMS, INC.
1300 N. McDowell Blvd.
Petaluma, CA 94954-1180
800-242-2376

SAFEGUARD BUSINESS SYSTEMS, INC.
455 Maryland Drive
Fort Washington, PA 19034
800-523-2422

AMES COLOR-FILE
12 Park Street
P.O. Box 120
Somerville, MA 02143-0120
800-343-2040

TAB PRODUCTS CO.
1400 Page Mill Road
Palo Alto, CA 94303
800-672-3109 (ext. 3304)

The medication list should include all medications including nonprescription and nontraditional remedies. If this list is available elsewhere it may not need to be regenerated.

UPDATING THE CHART

Patients' charts are never complete until a patient dies or stops receiving care from a practice. Thus, their contents and problem lists are ever changing. As the charts grow they become increasingly accurate records for patients. Because information should never be removed from the chart, mechanisms must be developed to allow for constant evolution in a patient's problem list. In the example on page 109, the "start" and

FIGURE 1. PHARMACEUTICAL CARE DATA SHEET

Pharmaceutical Care Record

Name Mary Blythe	DOB 7/10/62	Allergies NKDA,* Dogs, Cats, Dust, Grass, Pollen

Medical Problem List				Medication List				
Date		No.	Problem	Date		Prob #	Drug and Str.	Dose
Active	Resolved			Start	Stop			
–12/96		A	Depression	–9/97		A	Serzone 150 mg	BID
? <1980		B	Allergic Rhinitis	–6/97		B & A	Benadryl 25 mg	4 HS
		C		–1/97		B	Vancenase AQ	2 BID
		D		–6/97		B	Afrin	2 BID
		E		?			APAP	PRN HA
		F						
		G						
		H						
		I						
		J						
		K						
		L						
		M						
		N						
		O						
		P						
		Q						
		R						
		S						

Drug Therapy Problem List

Date		No.	Drug Therapy Problem with Description
Identified	Resolved		
12/29/97		1	Inappropriate compliance – overuse of Afrin and underuse of Vancenase AQ
12/29/97		2	Adverse drug reaction – nasal congestion from overuse of Afrin
12/29/97		3	Adverse drug reaction – nasal congestion and hypotension possibly due to Serzone
12/29/97		4	Dosage too high – dose and duration of Benadryl
		5	
		6	
		7	
		8	
		9	
		10	
		11	
		12	
		13	
		14	

Copyright 1994, Iowa Center for Pharmaceutical Care

*NKDA: No known drug allergies.

FIGURE 2. PHARMACEUTICAL CARE FLOW SHEET

DATES								
Test								

"stop" columns in the "medication list" section are used to continually update the list without removing information. If the list becomes unwieldy because of the number of changes made, a new list can be created and dated to supersede the old list. (Care should always be taken in the transcription process to avoid making errors in the new problem list—or in any other document in the chart.) The old list then goes behind the new one or into an archival portion of the chart. The new list becomes the only place to look for pertinent information on current problems.

FLOW SHEETS

Flow sheets are often included in patient charts to present data compactly or to make it easier to interpret over time. Weight, blood pressure, pulse, and other vital signs may be easier to follow if recorded in a table. Various doses of a drug, physical findings, and laboratory results may also be easier to track and analyze when presented in a table. Entire courses of disease management can often be documented for months or years on a single page of a well-designed flow sheet. An example of a flow sheet appears on page 110.

OTHER SECTIONS

Depending on the particular practice, the patient population, and the information collected, other sections may be necessary in the chart. For example, a separate section for laboratory reports may be needed so the provider does not have to sift through the whole chart to find them. Another section might contain records generated outside the pharmacy, such as hospitalization reports, physician records, and public or home health nursing reports. Correspondence, both incoming and outgoing, can make up another section. The correspondence section might include letters or faxes to and from physicians, other health care providers, caregivers, or insurance companies. It also could include a copy of the release signed by the patient or legal representative that authorizes pharmacists' correspondence with other parties. Requirements vary according to the individual practice; it is up to each pharmacy to decide what to include in the chart.

PROBLEM-ORIENTED CONTENT

Problem-oriented notes form the substance of the patient chart. They let the pharmacist know what information was considered in evaluating the patient's drug therapy, how the data were evaluated, details of the care plan, steps taken to date to implement the plan, outcome measures to be assessed, and the schedule for completing outcome assessments.

Each note is written about a single problem, or about a closely related group of problems, regarding the disease state or medication involved. The problems "inappropriate duration—5-day treatment with penicillin for strep throat" and "undesirable effect—constipation due to iron supplementation" would best be handled with two separate notes, because they are unrelated. In contrast, the problems "inappropriate duration—5-day treatment with penicillin for strep throat" and "need for additional drug therapy—untreated pain due to strep throat" are related and could be efficiently documented in one note. If the patient assessment reveals no drug therapy problems, a note stating "no drug therapy problems identified" should be written that contains the information leading to that conclusion and the plans for re-evaluation.

> ## CONFIDENTIALITY
>
> Confidentiality of the patient's pharmacy records must be guarded carefully. Within the pharmacy, a system should be in place to ensure the security of patient records, whether they are computerized or on paper. Firm policies should govern which pharmacy staff have access to patient charts, and in what capacity. The pharmacists and the pharmacy staff must understand that information in the record is to be provided to others only when authorized by the patient in writing (see the Authorization to Release Medical Information form on page 44) or when required by law. The confidentiality issue is especially important as pharmacists seek payment for services through third party payers.

Each note should be dated. If multiple entries are made on the same day, record the time the care was delivered. Each note should also be titled with the drug therapy problem it discusses. This title should be the same as that used on the problem list. If more than one problem is covered in a note, all drug therapy problems it discusses should be included in the title.

Some pharmacists may prefer to title a note with the medical problem it discusses, especially if they regularly share records with physicians or other health care professionals who are accustomed to the medical-problem format. The way the notes are titled is less important than using a consistent approach.

SOAP NOTES

The notes in the chart should be structured in a consistent format. The SOAP format, which is widely used in health care, is an excellent choice because other health care professionals can read and comprehend SOAP notes at a glance. SOAP is an acronym that stands for Subjective, Objective, Assessment, and Plan. Each term relates to a section of the note that contains a specific type of information. Developing a consistent approach to writing these notes helps pharmacists provide efficient care to patients.

The subjective and objective portions contain information from the patient, from exams performed, and from laboratory tests. This information serves as the basis or justification for the assessment and plan chosen for a new problem. It also describes the interim and current status of patients on follow-up.

The assessment and the plan should be a quick read and should convey what the provider believed was going on with the patient, what was done on that date, and the plans for both that date and for follow-up.

Subjective Information

The subjective section of the note is for recording information obtained from the patient or caregiver, or historical information that may not be known objectively. Only include information pertinent to specific drug therapy problems that the note discusses. Material that should go in this section includes:

- Patient's history of present illness (HPI),
- Past medical history (PMH),
- Social or family history (SH or FH),
- Allergies,
- Previous adverse drug reactions (ADR),
- Review of systems (ROS).

This section should also specify the medications involved in the problem being discussed and should explain how the patient is taking those medications.

Objective Information

The objective part of the note documents data collected about the patient that can be measured objectively, such as:

- Vital signs,
- Laboratory test results (from the original tests, not patient history),
- Findings from other tests,
- Physical examination results from a trained examiner.

Indicating who generated the objective data, and the date, may be appropriate. For example: "Physical exam 7/20/97 by Dr. Smith indicated HEENT [head, eye, ear, nose, and throat] exam WNL [within normal limits]."

THE ASSESSMENT

The assessment part of the note allows pharmacists to document what they feel is the current status of the problems discussed. The assessment should be based on data contained in the subjective and objective sections. The assessment will resemble the title of the note but will elaborate a bit on the problems rather than simply restating them. When a problem is first identified, the pharmacist may enter a brief description followed by the words "newly identified." When an assessment note is written after re-evaluating a problem—such as after a follow-up call—a straightforward way to indicate the assessment is to use terms such as "resolved" or "worsened." The assessment section is a good place to document special considerations or the rationale for the care plan, if such documentation seems necessary.

THE PLAN

The plan section is essentially a record of what a pharmacist did or plans to do for the patient, such as providing patient education or making recommendations to the patient, physician, or caregiver. Sufficient detail should be used so that the recommendations and how they will be implemented are clear to the reader. It should also be obvious whether the action has already been taken or is still being considered. The pharmacist may want to separate the portion of the plan that discusses action taken or planned from the portion that indicates how outcomes of the recommendations will be monitored. Physicians often separate their plans into diagnostic (Dx), therapeutic (Tx), and follow-up (F/U); pharmacists may wish to do the same.

Follow-up is an important part of the plan. In his book *Knowledge Coupling: New Premises and New Tools for Medical Care and Education,* Lawrence Weed discusses the importance of developing a mechanism for following up each problem identified:[3]

> Faulty understanding and defective decisions may be expected at the outset of a new case. Indeed, they are inevitable in the face of multiple variables. But failure to follow-up rigorously the results of those decisions is inexcusable. Action without follow-up is arrogance, especially where the objects of that action are living systems about which nothing is completely understood and in which conditions never remain fixed.

The F/U should include the interval planned before follow-up is necessary, the monitoring parameters that will be assessed at that time, and what will be done with that data. For example:

> F/U: Call patient in 3 weeks, assess ibuprofen effectiveness in relief of arthritis symptoms, any nausea/dyspepsia, changes in stool color. If arthritis improved and no ADR would continue at present dose F/U

again in 1 month. If no apparent ADR and Sx [symptoms] not relieved would call Dr. and recommend dosage increase to ibuprofen 600 mg QID [four times daily]. If ADR consider different dose or drug.

It is often helpful to document contingency plans if one has already spent time thinking about them, so that effort does not have to be repeated. The pharmacist should be able to read the plan and know exactly what happened and what is intended next. Furthermore, a colleague should be able to read, interpret, and act on the plan if the recording pharmacist is not available.

The desired therapeutic outcome (relief of arthritis symptoms) and possible negative outcomes that are anticipated (nausea/dyspepsia, changes in stool color) are placed in the follow-up part of the plan because these are parameters to be monitored. Also, the follow-up section is often the best place to document the patient's therapeutic goals since the pharmacist will determine whether goals have been met as part of the follow-up.

NEW NOTES FOR NEW PROBLEMS

After the SOAP note is written, it should be signed by the author— that is, the provider giving the care documented in the note. When the patient receives subsequent care, a new SOAP note should be generated for each problem addressed. This is a better approach than attaching addenda to previously generated notes. Follow-up notes are often short, and only need to cover changes and developments occurring between care episodes. Using a consistent format for the notes promotes efficiency as well as easier interpretation of the record by others, including physicians. Adhering to a standard format also helps pharmacists to quickly locate data they wish to present to patients and health care providers, thus saving time and subtly underscoring the pharmacist's professionalism.

The pharmacist's ability to write SOAP notes and keep good records improves with practice. Providing quality care and documenting it for all to see brings pharmacists one step closer to being integral members of the health care team.

CASE STUDY

Below are examples of SOAP notes written for Mary Blythe's problems, which were discussed in Chapters 4 and 5. More than one drug therapy problem is included in one note. The Pharmaceutical Care Data Sheet on page 109 is filled in with Mary's problem list. Abbreviations used in the case study are defined on page 118.

Mary Blythe

12/29/97

Inappropriate compliance — overuse of Afrin Nasal Spray and underuse of Vancenase AQ

Adverse drug reaction — nasal congestion from overuse of Afrin

S: *New Pt. to pharmacy requests Afrin Spray in addition to Rx for Serzone. She requests help in breathing better. Complains of increased allergy symptoms including nasal congestion and sinus problems for the last year since moving here, with continuous problems since then. States she has had allergy problems for "years" and is allergic to "just about everything—dogs, cats, dust, grasses, pollens." Was prescribed Vancenase AQ 2 sprays each nostril BID, but only uses PRN when severe congestion, and she doesn't feel it helps much. Uses Afrin Nasal Spray 2 sprays in each nostril twice daily for months, also uses Benadryl 100 mg @ HS for allergies and sleep. She feels the Afrin helps some and possibly also the Benadryl. She has never gotten "allergy shots." She quit smoking 2 years ago.*

O: *None*

A: *Inappropriate use of Afrin likely causing rebound congestion and aggravation of allergy symptoms.*

Lack of use of Vancenase resulting in ineffective treatment of nasal allergy symptoms.

P: *Counseled Mary on the consequences of overuse of Afrin and underuse of Vancenase AQ. Instructed her to use Afrin no more than twice daily and to alternate nostrils for each dose for 1 week, then reduce to NMT once daily and continue to alternate nostrils for the second week. She can then discontinue use. If Afrin needed in the future for congestion, she was instructed to use NMT once per day, in only one nostril, and for not more than 3 days. Mary agreed to try the Vancenase AQ on a regular basis after discussion of mechanism and efficacy, and patient was given a dosing reminder calendar to check off doses used. Inhaler technique tested after counseling and was appropriate.*

CASE STUDY

F/U: Call patient at home in one week. Assess Vancenase AQ compliance, status of Afrin use, and relief of nasal symptoms. Check on ADR from Vancenase, especially nasal dryness or irritation. If no change or worsening in symptoms or patient unable to tolerate Afrin taper, will then refer to physician for medical evaluation.

A. Pharmacist, R.Ph.

Adverse drug reaction — nasal congestion and hypotension possibly due to Serzone

S: See above. Additionally patient has been on Serzone 150 mg BID for 3 months for treatment of depression that has been ongoing for "about a year." She states that she is feeling much better and the Serzone has "been a lifesaver." She would like to continue on this medication due to the response she has seen. No complaints of HA, stomach upset, or drowsiness. Still some insomnia requiring Benadryl 100 mg at HS which seems to help. States she feels dizzy occasionally, especially on standing up. This has been more of a problem the last few months. BP in doctor's office runs "110/70 most of the time."

O: BP: 90/60 mm Hg, Pulse: 78 bpm

A: Serzone through alpha-receptor blocking effects could be contributing to both nasal congestion and hypotension. Although the hypotension is an unusual side effect with this medication, it is temporally associated with the initiation of this med in Mary.

P: Discussed the potential for the Serzone to be contributing to symptoms with Mary. Agreed with Mary not to recommend to her physician that Serzone be changed at this time. Letter written to physician making him aware of BP, potential connection with depression therapy, Mary's desire to continue therapy, and proposed follow-up plan.

F/U: When talk with patient in one week, assess depression status, change in nasal congestion, sleeping, and dizziness. Get BP readings if possible. If continued dizzy and hypotensive, refer to physician for assessment.

A. Pharmacist, R.Ph.

Dosage too high — dose and duration of Benadryl

S: Mary is taking Benadryl 100 mg @ HS for allergies and insomnia. She has taken this every night for months. She acknowledges that this may be a

CASE STUDY

residual symptom from her depression. Otherwise she feels well, has no problems with morning drowsiness, or complaints of dry mucosa, or other anti-cholinergic effects, and states she doesn't want to change her use of Benadryl at this time. She quit smoking 2 years ago, does not drink alcohol, and drinks 4-5 cups of decaf coffee per day.

O: *None*

A: *The dose and duration of Benadryl are inappropriate for the treatment of either allergies (not good 24-hour coverage) or insomnia (development of tolerance).*

P: *While Benadryl use is not optimal, it doesn't appear to be causing problems at present. Mary agrees to consider reducing its use if nasal congestion resolves. Counseled Mary on appropriate sleep hygiene and loaned her a set of relaxation tapes that she can try to see if they help her fall asleep. She agreed to buy a set if they help. When she is willing to try in the future, I instructed Mary that I would recommend decreasing the Benadryl dosage by 25 mg per night at weekly intervals. Once she is off, I would recommend taking NMT 50 mg at bedtime when her allergies are troublesome.*

F/U: *Discuss insomnia symptoms when call patient in 1 week. If nasal symptoms improving, reintroduce the thought of tapering off the Benadryl.*

A. Pharmacist, R.Ph.

GLOSSARY OF ABBREVIATIONS IN CASE STUDY

ADR: *adverse drug reaction*
BID: *twice daily*
BP: *blood pressure*
bpm: *beats per minute*
HA: *headache*

HS: *bedtime*
NMT: *no more than*
PRN: *as needed*
Pt: *patient*
Rx: *prescription*

REFERENCES

1. Weed LL. Medical records that guide and teach. *New Engl J Med.* 1968; 278:593-600.

2. Weed LL. Medical records that guide and teach. *New Engl J Med.* 1968;278:652-7.

3. Weed LL. *Knowledge Coupling: New Premises and New Tools for Medical Care and Education.* New York: Springer-Verlag; 1994:115.

Chapter 7

◆

Staffing Modifications for Pharmaceutical Care

Pharmacists consistently cite time constraints as a major obstacle to providing pharmaceutical care. Consequently, revamping the pharmacy work environment is a critical implementation strategy to assure that pharmacists are available for patient interactions. In many community pharmacies, efforts center on dispensing drugs efficiently, not on providing consultation services to patients. Typically the pharmacist's role is primarily to dispense drugs, handle phone calls to and from physicians, resolve drug-related problems as they present themselves, and answer customers' questions. To change from a practice oriented towards products to one that focuses on patients, as in pharmaceutical care, it is necessary first to systematically evaluate the pharmacy's operations, workflow, staff activities, and manpower requirements.

Bringing about comprehensive change in the work environment is often called "re-engineering," which Hammer and Champy define as "the fundamental rethinking and radical redesign of a business process to achieve dramatic improvements in critical measures of performance, such as cost, quality, service and speed."[1] The goal of re-engineering in a community pharmacy is to enhance operational efficiency by reassigning to nonpharmacists those dispensing tasks that do not require professional judgment. This frees the pharmacist to focus on the patient, yet minimizes the addition of new staff. By redefining the pharmacist's activities and applying simple mathematical analysis, operations can be assessed in a wide range of practice environments.

IDENTIFYING WORK ACTIVITIES

Identifying and categorizing all the work activities currently occurring in the pharmacy should be done first when attempting to change or improve on existing processes. Examples of these activities include:

- Services related to dispensing prescription medications,
- Drug product purchasing and inventory control,
- Merchandising of items that are not health related,
- Customer relations,
- Budgeting,
- Planning,
- Sales and marketing.

Since prescription dispensing is likely to be the major activity occupying pharmacists' time, it is best to begin by analyzing the steps involved in preparing and distributing medications to patients. The dispensing process is amazingly similar from one pharmacy to the next and essentially progresses through a series of activities performed by pharmacists and technicians. By examining each step and asking how things are done, why they are done a certain way, and who is the best person to perform each task, alternative approaches will begin to emerge.

FIGURE 1. PHARMACY WORKFLOW FOR DISPENSING-RELATED ACTIVITIES

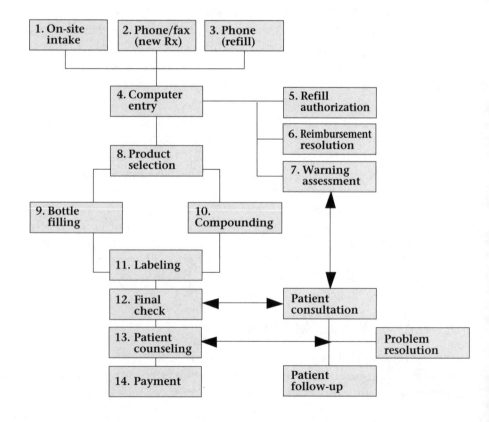

As Figure 1 shows, the typical prescription dispensing process begins with a request for medication, which is communicated either in person, by telephone, or by fax (steps 1, 2, and 3, respectively). All three intake routes may be handled by any or all staff members. Differentiating the various intake methods allows for later reassigning responsibility to appropriate staff.

Once the request has been received, the new or refill prescription is usually entered into the computer (step 4) and is processed. The following problems can prevent computer processing from being completed:

- No refills remain on the prescription, which means that authorization must be sought from the prescriber (step 5).

- A reimbursement problem needs to be resolved with the payer (step 6).

- The dispensing software generates a warning about a drug interaction, duplication, or allergy (step 7).

While the information is entered into the computer, or immediately afterwards, the product is selected (step 8), the bottle is filled (step 9), or the product is compounded (step 10). Appropriate labels (step 11) are then prepared and applied to the dispensing container. A final check (step 12) to assure accuracy and legal adherence is performed before the product is given to the patient. After the patient is counseled about the medication's use and side effects (step 13) and pays the pharmacy (step 14), he or she leaves with the prescription medication.

When the process is delineated this way, individual steps can be delegated to other staff members so that the pharmacist is freed for direct patient-care activities, which are depicted on the right-hand side of the figure (patient consultation, patient follow-up, and problem resolution). However, delegation can only occur if the fundamental roles of everyone involved are clearly defined and agreed upon.

REDEFINING ROLES

Redefining the role of the pharmacist and of supportive personnel in the pharmacy can be very difficult. Inherent to the process is the need to challenge existing paradigms about pharmacists, pharmacy, and professional responsibility to patients. Although the role of the pharmacist in a given setting depends somewhat on the operational needs of the pharmacy, in a pharmaceutical care practice it must be focused on professional activities that address patients' drug therapy needs. Daily operations management by the pharmacist should be minimized to allow for uninterrupted patient interaction.

In the re-engineered pharmacy, the primary responsibility of the pharmacist shifts from dispensing drugs to providing patient care. The time freed up by delegating dispensing tasks is replaced with activities in which the pharmacist interacts directly with patients and handles tasks legally mandated by the state in which the pharmacist practices. At a minimum, the pharmacist must retain responsibility for:

- Verifying the accuracy of dispensed products,
- Doing prospective drug utilization review as defined by the Omnibus Budget Reconciliation Act of 1990 (OBRA '90),
- Patient counseling.

All other tasks related to the dispensing workflow should be delegated to trained technicians.

Technician roles need to be modified significantly as well, although how much they change in each pharmacy depends on how involved in dispensing the technicians already are. For pharmacists to be able to focus on patient interaction, technicians must be given the tools and authority to maintain the product dispensing workflow up to the point where the pharmacist verifies the prescription and delivers the medication to the patient. Except for step 7, warning assessment, a technician or clerk should assume responsibility for everything from prescription intake to product labeling.

ESTIMATING PERSONNEL NEEDS

After identifying a pharmacy's operational elements, the relative contribution in each area by pharmacists versus nonpharmacist staff must be determined. Since sophisticated time studies are cost-prohibitive for most community pharmacies, an alternative approach is to estimate the percentage contribution by various staff to individual tasks. Soliciting input from both pharmacists and support personnel will enhance the estimate's accuracy.

To begin, staff members should come to agreement on what percent of the time each dispensing-related task is performed by either a pharmacist, technician, or clerk. In the example represented by Table 1, on-site intake is performed 60% of the time by a pharmacist, 20% by a technician, and 20% by a clerk.

Once each task has been evaluated and the percentages of time recorded, the relative contributions currently made by each staff category can be determined. Total the individual task percentages in the "current" column for each of the three staff categories and divide by the total possible percent (in this case, divide by 1400 because 14 tasks are listed) to get each staff category's relative contribution to dispensing. Table 1 shows that an estimated 64% of dispensing-related activities in the example are being performed by pharmacists, while technicians and clerks contribute

TABLE 1. STAFFING ADJUSTMENT WORKSHEET

Dispensing Task	% Pharmacist (Current)	% Pharmacist (Desired)	% Technician (Current)	% Technician (Desired)	% Clerk (Current)	% Clerk (Desired)
On-site intake	60	0	20	20	20	80
Phone/fax intake	95	10	5	90	0	0
Phone refills	20	5	75	90	5	5
Computer entry	90	0	10	90	0	10
Refill authorization	75	0	25	95	0	5
Reimbursement resolution	75	20	25	80	0	0
Warning assessment	100	100	0	0	0	0
Product selection	20	0	75	95	5	5
Bottle filling	20	0	75	95	5	5
Compounding	65	10	35	90	0	0
Labeling	75	0	25	95	0	5
Final check	100	100	0	0	0	0
Patient counseling	100	100	0	0	0	0
Payment	0	0	60	10	30	90
Relative Contribution	64	25	31	61	5	15
	Pharmacist Hours/Week	Pharmacist Hours/Week	Technician Hours/Week	Technician Hours/Week	Clerk Hours/Week	Clerk Hours/Week
Calculated Dispensing Hours	96	37	46	91	7	22

31% and 5%, respectively. Once the current percentages are clear, the challenge is shifting pharmacists' contribution to either technicians or clerks.

To begin re-engineering, each individual task must be evaluated and responsibility reassigned, in keeping with the professional roles of the new pharmaceutical care paradigm. Before the "desired" columns in Table 1 can be filled in, the pharmacy staff needs to discuss who is the best person to perform a given task and how certain tasks should be split. Then a goal percentage contribution for each task should be assigned to the pharmacists, technicians, and clerks. The Table 1 example illustrates goals of having pharmacists perform no on-site intake, clerks 80%, and technicians 20%. In the scenario that the table represents, the patient would be greeted by the clerk, the prescription request would be given to the technician, and the pharmacist would devote his or her time to interacting with the patient on drug therapy matters.

After goal percentages are assigned for each task, the figures should be tallied in the "desired" columns of Table 1 and divided by 1400 (again, because there are 14 dispensing tasks) to yield the relative contribution desired by each staff category. The table shows that the desired contributions to dispensing are 25% for pharmacists, 61% for technicians, and 15% for clerks.

To translate the relative contribution percentages to calculated dispensing hours (which appear in the bottom row of Table 1), it is necessary to do an intermediate calculation based on each staff member's estimates of the number of hours spent in dispensing tasks. These figures are shown in Table 2.

TABLE 2. ESTIMATED CURRENT DISPENSING HOURS

Staffing Category	Total Staffing Hours/Week	Dispensing Hours/Week
Pharmacist	165	100
Technician	60	40
Clerk	40	10
Total	**265**	**150**

To fill out Table 2, each staff person should provide his or her best estimates of actual hours spent on dispensing-related tasks. One way to do that is to take the total hours worked per week and subtract the estimated amount of time spent on inventory maintenance, management, cleaning, or other tasks that are not specifically identified on the Staffing Adjustment Worksheet in Table 1. The time that remains after subtracting nondispensing tasks should be totaled for each staff category and then plugged in to the "dispensing hours/week" column in Table 2. The table shows that, in this example, an estimated 100 pharmacist hours, 40 technician hours, and 10 clerk hours—a total of 150 hours—are devoted to dispensing-related tasks each week.

To estimate new manpower requirements, multiply the total estimated dispensing hours in Table 2 by the current and desired percentages in Table 1. For example, since the goal is for 61% of those 150 hours to be contributed by technician staff, 150 x .61 = 91.5 hours per week. (In Table 1 the number is rounded to 91.) That is an increase of more than 40 hours over the estimated current contribution of 40 hours, which means that additional technician staff must be hired or duties of existing staff must be reassigned. Next, similar calculations should be performed for clerk hours and pharmacist hours. In Table 1, the results of these calculations are shown in the last row, titled "calculated dispensing hours."

The number of calculated pharmacist dispensing hours per week minus the pharmacist dispensing hours desired per week (both shown in the bottom row of Table 1) reveals the number of hours that pharmacists would be freed up for patient care activities: 96 - 37 = 59.

STAFFING ADJUSTMENTS

After the total number of additional dispensing hours have been calculated for the technician and clerk categories, it is necessary to make decisions regarding staff scheduling and hiring. Although reassigning duties to existing staff is one option, realistically it is likely that other staff will need to be hired to perform their previous duties. In any event, the staffing adjustments will probably require the addition of at least some staffing hours to the budget.

If man-hours must be added, the optimal approach would be to allocate them to nonskilled activities that can be performed by workers earning the lowest wage. For example, a technician whose hourly wage is twice the minimum set by the government spends 50% of his time dispensing and 50% of his time cleaning shelves and checking in inventory. If the cleaning and inventory tasks are assigned to a nonskilled worker who can be paid minimum wage, the cost is half what it would be if another technician were hired at the higher pay rate to perform dispensing functions. The exact times that the new hours will be added should be decided after carefully considering workload needs.

STAFF TRAINING

While the pharmacists are developing their pharmaceutical care skills, technicians and clerical staff must also be trained to perform new functions. Only through adequate training and experience will the staff gain the confidence to assume greater responsibility for product dispensing. Careful planning for staff development is critical to re-engineering success.

What then, are the essential training elements to be considered? Using tasks outlined in the dispensing workflow (Figure 1) as a guide, the preparedness of existing or new staff to perform each task should be assessed. After each staff member's baseline skills have been determined, a schedule for addressing individual staff members' training needs should be outlined. It may take weeks or months for new staff, or even existing staff, to be ready to perform computer entry tasks, handle compounding procedures, solve reimbursement problems, or—if permitted by the state practice act—receive a prescription order over the telephone. Written policies and procedures describing how staff should perform various tasks will facilitate the training process. Using quality assurance measures will help maintain customer service and satisfaction.

Do not assume that pharmacists must train all technicians and clerical staff themselves. Using peer-training methods is very effective. Existing staff members already have considerable expertise that they can use to mentor new employees or other existing staff. Appropriate use of everyone's talents and abilities will build teamwork and enhance buy-in to the newly defined practice.

> **QUALIFICATIONS FOR TECHNICAL STAFF**
>
> - Good interpersonal skills,
> - Detail oriented,
> - Quick to learn new skills and concepts,
> - Can deal with the stress of a demanding workload.
>
> Additionally, for technicians who will process prescriptions:
>
> - Able to read and interpret physician orders,
> - Knowledge of drug names,
> - Familiar with pharmacy billing methods,
> - Computer literate,
> - Above average aptitude for math,
> - Professional appearance,
> - Ability to work independently,
> - Technician certification or medical training background.

In conjunction with staff training, it is necessary to develop appropriate job descriptions so that staff members fully understand the new roles and functions. Using the dispensing tasks listed in Table 1 as a guide, one can assign primary and secondary responsibility for each task to individuals or to specific positions. Job descriptions not only facilitate training and evaluation, but they also convey clear expectations, which enhances efficiency by minimizing duplicate effort. A key example is uncertainty regarding who should answer the telephone and when. By assigning primary, secondary, and perhaps even tertiary responsibility, individuals can reasonably predict when it is necessary for them to answer the phone—which avoids having several staffers' thoughts and movements directed toward the phone at the same time.

STAFF RECRUITMENT

Key skill areas need to be considered when the decision is made to reassign or hire technical staff. Since all staff members interact with customers either in person or by telephone, interpersonal skills are essential. At the same time, the individual should be detail oriented, quick to learn new skills and concepts, and able to cope with the stress of time constraints and a demanding workload. Technicians who will process prescriptions must be able to read and interpret physician orders, be knowledgeable about drug names, and understand pharmacy billing methods. They should also be computer literate and have above-average math aptitude. Finally, a professional appearance and the ability to work independently are important.

To attract talented individuals who can fulfill the expectations set forth in the re-engineered staffing plan, compensation must be appropriate. Remember, what this person is able to accomplish will determine whether the pharmacist has time to provide pharmaceutical care. It is preferable to search for experienced technicians with certification credentials. If they are not available, other persons with a medical background should be sought. In all cases, a confident, intelligent, and motivated person is absolutely necessary. At all costs, avoid recruitment efforts that do not explicitly detail the job requirements.

REFERENCE

1. Hammer M, Champy J. *Reengineering the Corporation: A Manifesto for Business Revolution.* New York: Harper Collins; 1993.

Chapter 8

◆

Re-engineering the Pharmacy Layout

The layout of traditional community pharmacies is geared toward achieving the highest possible sales volume at the lowest possible cost. Typically pharmacies try to maximize front-end store traffic, encourage point-of-sale purchases, and minimize losses due to theft and breakage. The prescription department—set off from the rest of the store in a dominant position at the rear—may be elevated from the general selling floor and may display impulse or high-margin items near the register. An auxiliary service, such as a post office or package shipping service, may be located nearby. The counter is designed so prescriptions can be dropped off, picked up, and paid for efficiently. A separate patient waiting area and patient counseling area may already be in place, although quite likely they are only partially functional. Figure 1 depicts a typical community pharmacy layout before it has been redesigned for pharmaceutical care.

The re-engineered pharmacy is designed around a "health care center" concept, in which tasks and materials related to patient care are grouped as close together as possible. For the re-engineered pharmacy to be conducive to patient care, barriers to patient interaction must be avoided. Creating private areas in which the pharmacist and patient can get together and talk, known as consultation areas, is a good way to promote effective interaction. Introducing a consultation area to the pharmacy is not terribly difficult. Equally important—but probably harder to do—is incorporating new design elements that help change the pharmacist's workflow habits and patients' expectations.

FIGURE 1. PHARMACY LAYOUT BEFORE REDESIGN

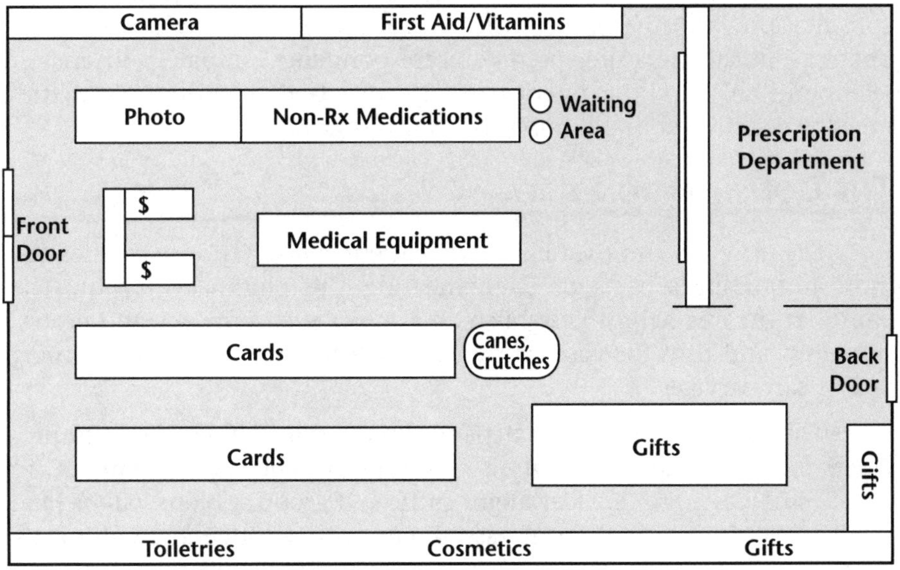

THE OBJECTIVES OF A REDESIGN

At a minimum, when a facility is redesigned for pharmaceutical care the objectives should be:

- Facilitating the provision of care,
- Enhancing the health care image of the pharmacy,
- Maintaining or improving workflow,
- Minimizing disruptions from patient traffic,
- Maximizing the use of space.

Each individual pharmacy operation will need to assess its current work environment to create a redesign plan consistent with available resources. The pharmacy must also evaluate the design's effectiveness and be prepared for continued change as the pharmacist's role in patient care evolves and patients' expectations expand.

Early on, the pharmacy staff needs to clearly define the patient care process that will be carried out at the pharmacy. How will the steps of collecting and evaluating data, formulating and implementing care plans, and following up with patients translate to actual pharmacist activities? And, more important, what type of environment is best suited to accomplish them?

Since the data collection process can only be successful if a professional relationship is established with the patient, an area must be available where the pharmacist can meet with the patient to collect data confidentially and free from distractions. Following the patient consultation, the pharmacist will need a place to review medical and pharmaceutical literature, prepare correspondence, initiate and answer telephone calls, and document patient care activities. All these activities must be considered in planning the new design.

THE CONSULTATION AREA

Creating a semiprivate area for patient consultation is one of the most important aspects of re-engineering the pharmacy layout. The consultation area helps to establish an atmosphere of privacy and professionalism and thus increases patients' awareness that they are receiving health care services.

The area's specific design depends on the scope of services to be provided and their expected volume. For typical patient consultations, an area as small as 50 square feet might suffice. If group sessions will be held or services involving physical assessment will be offered, significantly larger areas may be needed to accommodate extra people, furniture, and supplies.

A busy pharmacy with several pharmacists on duty may need more than one consultation area if two or more patient care encounters will occur simultaneously. Regardless of the number of patient consultation areas or their size, some key features should be considered.

LOCATION

The consultation area should be strategically located to allow easy access by both pharmacists and patients. Since pharmacists will need to continue to oversee dispensing functions and supervise technicians, they must be able to interact with patients in the same general area. A consultation area connected to the pharmacy dispensing area, as shown in Figure 2, allows the pharmacist to check prescriptions and then enter the consultation area to talk with a patient without walking very far. The tasks for prescription processing should occur in a single direction—from the intake window to the spot where the pharmacist does the final check—to keep staff from colliding and to prevent duplication of effort.

The nonprescription medications and health-related items should be located near the patient waiting and patient consultation areas. This way pharmacists can easily identify patients who require assistance and they do not have to walk a long distance to retrieve products needed during a patient consultation.

FIGURE 2. PHARMACY LAYOUT AFTER REDESIGN

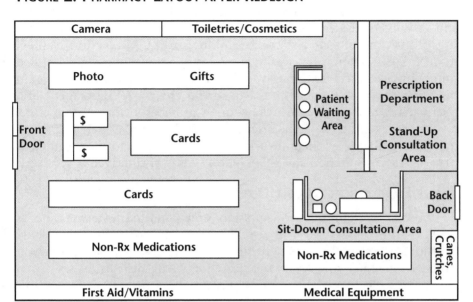

It is best to locate the consultation area away from the cash register to avoid the noise, traffic, and lack of privacy of a point-of-sale location. Whether the pharmacist should be involved in monetary transactions is open to debate and is certainly a site-specific consideration. However, if at all possible, operational policies should be initiated that require the patient to pay for prescriptions at a location away from the consultation area, as is common in other medical service operations.

SITTING OR STANDING

Should the consultation area be designed so that pharmacists interact with patients while sitting down, or standing? The decision should be made after carefully evaluating some key issues. First, if the majority of patients are elderly, will they find it difficult to stand for extended periods? Will some patients interpret not being able to sit down as an indication that the pharmacist doesn't really have time to spend with them? If only one pharmacist is on duty at a given time, will sitting to talk with a patient and then repeatedly standing up to supervise dispensing functions cause excessive fatigue for the pharmacist?

Some pharmacists have designed elevated counseling areas that allow them to sit while checking prescriptions and talking with patients. The patient typically stands at a lower level than the pharmacist, who can maintain eye contact on the same level even though the patient is standing on the floor below. This arrangement may be useful for dealing with the majority of patients.

The pharmacist should consider whether space is available for both options. Figure 2 depicts a stand-up area for shorter counseling sessions and a sit-down area for extended consultations. This allows for maximum flexibility; the pharmacist can individualize the interaction to meet specific patient circumstances. In some cases, a single area could be used simply by placing a waist-high work counter, such as a short bookcase, in the same semiprivate area with a desk and chairs. While patient and pharmacist stand side by side, the counter provides a work surface and a place to put items that will be discussed with the patient, such as medications or health-related literature. It is always advisable to allow sufficient space in the consultation area to include a spouse or caregiver, if necessary.

SINGLE FUNCTION OR DOUBLE DUTY?

When designing a consultation area, another consideration is whether the pharmacist will use the space to complete care-related functions after the direct patient interaction is over. The ideal situation would be to have one work area for supervising dispensing tasks and being available to patients, and a private office for detailed cognitive work, but this is not always possible. In a pharmacy where only one pharmacist is on duty at a time—who therefore needs to be easily accessible—it may be necessary to create care plans and do other work that requires concentration in the same space where consultations are held. If so, the consultation area will need to be equipped with a desk, computer, telephone, reference books, and other resources.

COMMUNICATING THE RIGHT MESSAGE

In creating a space to provide patient care, it is critical that the environment clearly communicates the message that "this pharmacy is a place to receive health care services." All too often, patients receive a conflicting message that the pharmacy is primarily focused on selling products. A good way to evaluate the subliminal message being delivered in the pharmacy is to go outside and approach the front door as a customer would. While entering and walking through the pharmacy, the pharmacist should take note of what comes into view and what it suggests.

- What is the first thing a person notices when walking through the door?
- Are there health-related cues, or is most of the merchandise commonly found in a grocery, hardware, or convenience store?
- Does the overall environment focus on products, or does it suggest that the patient is the focus?
- What evidence exists that the pharmacy staff cares about patient comfort and health?

Although items that are not health related might, by necessity, be part of the inventory mix, the pharmacist should ensure that health-related items and services are separate and prominently displayed in an area that suggests a medical focus. (Note how the merchandise is rearranged in Figure 2 as compared with Figure 1.)

Among other things to consider is whether the pharmacy is neat, clean, and well maintained. If it is dirty, cluttered, or needs repair, patients may think that a less-than-professional service is offered at the pharmacy. Are patients greeted when they enter? Are their needs assessed? Do they know what to expect when they enter the prescription department? If not, patients may feel that they are not the focus of what happens in the pharmacy.

THE WAITING AREA

Think about other health care environments the patient may frequent. Almost everyone has been in a hospital or physician's office and therefore equates health care with a quiet, comfortable, and clean environment. There is usually a receptionist to greet and direct patients and a designated waiting area with indirect lighting. A calming, quiet waiting area is especially important for patients who do not feel well or are in pain. These same patients may leave the physician's office and come straight to the pharmacy. If so, they should not be expected to wander the aisles waiting to be called; there should be a place for them to rest while their prescription is being prepared and while they wait for the pharmacist to speak with them.

The pharmacist should consider all aspects of the waiting area. Do the seats have arms to make getting in and out of the chair easier? Is the lighting too bright and potentially stimulating, or is it indirect and relaxing? To encourage patients to wait rather than demand immediate service, materials should be provided to occupy them. Health-related literature, videos, computer kiosks, and even children's toys help pass the time and convey a patient focus, while simultaneously enhancing the pharmacy's health care image. Patients may also appreciate complimentary refreshments such as decaffeinated coffee or tea, or sugar-free juices. Be sure they are healthful items so as not to encourage habits that the pharmacist may later have to counsel the patient to avoid.

TRAFFIC PATTERNS

The location of the waiting area and the patient consultation area must take into account current traffic patterns and patient habits. Although minimizing disruption of current traffic patterns is a good idea, changing them probably cannot be avoided altogether. It may be difficult, but it is not impossible to train patients to take alternate routes through the pharmacy, drop prescriptions in a new spot, and talk to a pharmacist in a totally different location than they are used to. Staff should help direct patients as appropriate and signage should be strategically placed to make it easier for patients to cooperate with the changes.

The waiting area should be close enough to the dispensing and consultation areas that patients do not have to walk long distances or call undue attention to themselves. To maintain privacy and prevent potential eavesdropping on conversations in the consultation area, the pharmacy should have background music or enough "white noise"—such as the hum of a soda machine or the sound of air conditioning—that other pharmacy customers cannot easily hear the counseling session.

Physical Re-engineering

Physically re-engineering the layout of the pharmacy does not necessarily require extensive or expensive changes. It is usually possible to work around the existing layout, making only slight changes to encourage a patient care atmosphere. While evaluating the current layout and considering potential changes, keep in mind the ease with which changes can be made, the potential disruptions they will cause, the cost of re-design, and how long changes will take.

Physical barriers that are impossible to eliminate, such as beams and pillars, should be identified. As much as possible, use physical barriers to their advantage: for example, a large pillar or support helps create a natural private space that could be transformed into a consultation area.

Locate semipermanent fixtures, such as water sources, electrical outlets, computer hookups, and phone jacks, and decide whether any changes are needed. Water accessibility is always important if laboratory assessments will be done or when hands-on patient contact will be made. Remember to think toward future needs and not just current plans for expansion to a pharmaceutical care practice. Although the number of electrical outlets may seem sufficient, they can quickly become over-loaded if you add computers or other electrical equipment; adding too many extension cords creates a fire hazard. Phone jacks are critical so that enough phones are available for conducting follow-up with patients and coordinating care with other providers.

Space limitations are a universal problem in pharmacies but they are not insurmountable. By carefully evaluating existing turnover and profit margins, as well as determining how specific products contribute to the professional and business mission, pharmacists can identify items to discontinue. After expendable merchandise is removed, fixtures and inventory can be rearranged to establish the "health care center" where the dispensing, waiting, and consultation areas are located. To make the design flexible, portable office partitions are used with great success in many pharmacies. Not only are they less costly than erecting permanent walls, but they allow areas to be expanded or adjusted to fit needs that were not originally anticipated. A standard six-foot height is recommended, although some pharmacies may have special needs that call for higher or lower walls. Glass partitions are also available that offer privacy but keep the consultation area visible, which some pharmacists consider a good marketing strategy. Other patients who see consultations taking place may ask for more information about the pharmacy's patient care services. Glass partitions may also be useful for security and liability reasons: they allow the pharmacist a view of the pharmacy floor, and they let others see that only professional activities are taking place in the consultation area.

The most important thing to remember when re-engineering the pharmacy layout is that the best configuration is one that meets a particular pharmacy's needs and budget. The goal is to establish a place to talk with patients privately without disrupting the workflow—and to do so in a way that projects a professional health care image.

Chapter 9

◆

Marketing
Pharmaceutical Care

Investing in building the capacity to supply pharmaceutical care services is critical, but equally important is investing in creating a *demand* for these services. In essence, pharmacy is developing a supply of pharmaceutical care services for a need it has identified in the health care system, a need that primarily results from negative health outcomes associated with drug therapy problems. Unfortunately, patients do not yet commonly recognize the value of pharmaceutical care and so they do not demand these services.

Knowing the product thoroughly and being able to match its features and benefits to a specific need is one of the most important elements in a successful marketing effort.

The marketing difficulties posed by lack of patient familiarity with this new service are compounded by pharmacists' limited experience with marketing. Very few pharmacists have education, training, or experience in developing a marketing plan or strategy. Most pharmacists have not had to actively market their services in the past and are uncomfortable in this role. Consequently, pharmacists are faced with the formidable challenge of re-engineering their practices to provide pharmaceutical care, while also initiating a marketing strategy to create demand for it. Pharmacists must build the demand and supply for pharmaceutical care services simultaneously.

This chapter outlines how to develop an effective pharmaceutical care marketing strategy and reviews techniques to make pharmacists more comfortable with the role of personal selling. The combination of personal selling skills and a detailed marketing strategy allows pharmacists to successfully promote and generate demand for their pharmaceutical care services.

APPLYING MARKETING PRINCIPLES TO PHARMACEUTICAL CARE

When marketing pharmaceutical care, the pharmacist must first realize that marketing a service differs from marketing a product. Because consumers cannot touch and examine a service to fully appreciate it, they must experience the service. Due to this limitation, service providers must focus their marketing efforts on fully describing the features and benefits of the service.[1,2] Accordingly, most patients, prescribers, and payers need to be educated about pharmaceutical care before they will understand its purposes and benefits.

The general framework for marketing follows four principles called the four P's: Product, Price, Promotion, and Place. A fifth P, Positioning, is also considered a factor.[2-4] Cooper discusses these marketing principles in the context of health care and refers to these elements as CAPS: Cost/Consideration (Price); Access/Availability (Place); Promotion; and Service Development (Product).[5] A blending of each of these components leads to a successful marketing mix.

> ### THE 'P'S' OF MARKETING
>
> Five principles should be considered in developing any marketing plan:
>
> - Product
> - Price
> - Promotion
> - Place
> - Position.

The first principle, Product, is simply the item marketed. In the case of pharmaceutical care, the product is actually a service. The pharmaceutical care service offered may be a general one aimed at resolving all drug therapy problems, or it may be a service specific to a disease state, such as diabetes.

Setting an appropriate Price, the second marketing principle, is important to the successful marketing of any new service. This is a source of particular frustration for pharmacists, since they have limited experience pricing their cognitive services. The pricing for services should be firmly established before any marketing begins. (Further exploration of pharmaceutical care pricing is described in Chapter 10.)

It is important to recognize that Promotion, the third principle, encompasses much more than advertising. Promotion also includes the publicity, public relations activities, and personal selling of the pharmaceutical care service. A description and comparison of the many types of promotions occurs later in this chapter.

Last, but not least, is Place in the marketing mix. Making the product available in the right place at the right time is important to any product, but particularly important to the success of pharmaceutical care. For example, a pharmacist may offer to provide pharmaceutical care at the employer's place of business, for the ease and convenience of employees.

A fifth P that is often included, Positioning, addresses how the product will be viewed in the minds of prospective patients. Positioning creates a niche or "want" for the service in the patient's mind. A marketing effort positions the pharmacist as a medication expert and the patient's partner in managing specific health care needs. By promoting a pharmaceutical care service with the image of meeting certain needs, pharmacists create a desire for the service in the minds of their patients.

IDENTIFYING CUSTOMERS

When developing a marketing strategy, it is critically important to identify the target markets for pharmaceutical care service. Target markets are groups of customers who behave in similar patterns.[2, 4-7] For example, a population of patients with diabetes would be targeted for a marketing initiative on a diabetes pharmaceutical care service. An attempt to market such a product to the general public would be cost-prohibitive and poorly rewarded. By identifying the members of the target market, a marketing plan is more efficiently and effectively focused to the appropriate population.

Pharmacists should also develop a list of stakeholders in their market area. A stakeholder is anyone who can affect the success of the pharmacy practice. Examples of stakeholders include other health care providers, employer groups,

---

ADOPTION CURVE

Understanding patient behavior helps pharmacists develop effective marketing strategies. Not all patients behave the same way. Past research on patient responses to new ideas identified the "Adoption Curve" as a description of patient behavior.[8]

Consumers	Percentages
Innovators	**2.5%**
Venturesome, take risks in trying new ideas	
Early adopters	**13.5%**
Opinion leaders, carefully evaluate new ideas	
Early majority	**34%**
Deliberate, rarely a leader	
Adopts sooner than average consumer	
Late majority	**34%**
Skeptical, adopts after the majority	
Late adopters	**16%**
Laggards, tradition bound, suspicious of innovation	

Pharmacists should identify the individual innovators and early adopters within their target market for initial marketing efforts. These are the people who are most likely to be open to trying a new service like pharmaceutical care. By selling pharmaceutical care services to the innovators and early adopters, pharmacists can enjoy early success, build their confidence, and have a business base for their practice.

third party payers, or health care brokers. Although these groups are not direct consumers of the product, they can and do have an effect on the practice. Before any marketing begins, listing the target markets and stakeholders is an important first step that helps guide the marketing action plan.

Pharmacists can learn more about their patients' behavior by holding patient focus groups. In focus groups, a representative sample of consumers is gathered together to discuss and share their views on an issue, idea, or proposal. This strategy, if done with an unbiased facilitator, helps uncover patient needs and desires for a new service and get feedback regarding a current pharmaceutical care service. Focus groups offer the secondary effect of informally marketing the pharmaceutical care service to the participants.

Pharmacists can also market to individual patients by determining their unmet health and medication needs through casual conversations. Although less efficient than focus groups, this one-to-one strategy helps pharmacists identify and target individual patients as potential candidates for specific pharmaceutical care services.

DEFINING THE PRODUCT

Pharmacists should identify pharmaceutical care products to develop based on an understanding of and response to the unmet needs of their pharmacy's particular patients or the local health care system. Based on these needs, pharmacists should consider what the local market will support, and avoid providing unnecessary or duplicated services. Pharmacists should decide if they will offer one or more of the following types of services: a general pharmaceutical care product, disease state management services, or ancillary services (e.g., monitoring of blood pressure, blood glucose, or cholesterol). Developing services targeted to the needs of the pharmacy's patient population makes marketing easier and more effective.

Once the types of pharmaceutical care services to be offered are identified, pharmacists must be able to describe them to patients, other health care providers, and third party payers. General descriptions, as shown in the box on page 140, can be useful.

Pharmacists also must determine the specific features of those services and be able to clearly describe them to their patients. Some examples of the features of pharmaceutical care include:

- Drug therapy assessment,
- Patient education and counseling,
- Ongoing medication management and monitoring,
- Disease state management services,
- Compliance counseling,

- Development of care plans,
- Specialized clinical/laboratory services,
- Counseling on nonprescription drugs,
- Communication with all other health care providers,
- A written report to the patient of all findings and recommendations.

Describing the features provides only half the marketing message to patients, however. They also need to know how the services benefit them. The pharmacist's perceptions about the value of pharmaceutical care may vary greatly from the patient's. Patients choose benefits that meet their individual perceived needs—and each patient's needs are different.

Part of the marketing success of pharmaceutical care is making the patient aware that pharmaceutical care is a new and innovative service that is very different from traditional pharmacy service. The pharmaceutical care service could be described as a more thorough, in-depth service that includes an extensive patient review and ongoing follow-up to ensure that health improvements occur. It offers patients a health care provider with the training, skills, and knowledge in drug therapy to provide this valuable service. It is important to assure patients that, although they have received good care in the past with traditional pharmacy, this care did not represent the extensive level of service now offered in pharmaceutical care.

PHARMACEUTICAL CARE IS...

- An informational partnership between patients and pharmacists.
- A collaborative process with physicians and other health care providers that ensures the patient achieves the desired health care outcome.
- A service that helps consumers better understand their health status and drug therapy so they can make more informed health care decisions.

BENEFITS OF PHARMACEUTICAL CARE

- It may save lives.
- It helps people become and stay healthier.
- It saves people money.
- It helps patients learn more about their health care.
- It makes patients better informed.
- It equips patients to make better decisions.
- It helps patients take charge of their health.
- It builds a trusting relationship between the patient, physician, and pharmacist.
- Patients may experience less loss of time from work due to illness.
- It reduces emergency room visits and unnecessary physician appointments due to preventable drug therapy problems.

These benefits demonstrate the value of pharmaceutical care to all potential stakeholders (patients, health care providers, employers, third party payers, etc.).

Targeting the Marketing Message

An important part of creating a marketing plan is developing a target message for each stakeholder. By matching features to benefits for each individual stakeholder, pharmacists can create concise, effective, and targeted messages. Knowing the product thoroughly and being able to match its features and benefits to a specific need is one of the most important elements in a successful marketing effort. As a tool, the chart shown in Figure 1 can be used to develop the features and benefits for each stakeholder.

The Fifteen-Second Commercial

Pharmacists should be able to quickly and clearly describe their services to stakeholders in a way that is sometimes called the "15-second commercial." Fifteen seconds is the amount of time pharmacists can expect to hold a potential patient's attention to describe a pharmaceutical care service. This brief description of the service should include three components:

- The product definition,
- An explanation of its benefits,
- The price.

Figure 1. Chart for Plotting Features and Benefits of Pharmaceutical Care

Stakeholder	Need	How Pharmaceutical Care Meets Need (Feature)	Benefit
Patients:			
New			
Existing			
Patient families and/or caretakers			
Physicians			
Third party payers			
Employers			
Others			

The product and its features should be described in terms readily understood by the patient, and its value or benefit to that person should be emphasized. The price should be presented in comparison with the service's terms and benefits.

All pharmacists and pharmacy staff should be familiar with the 15-second commercial technique and be able to use it with patients in the pharmacy. Writing out a script describing a particular service, discussing and identifying the type of patient who will benefit from the service, and having everyone practice using it helps individual staff members develop their own personal style and comfort with presenting the commercial. The following example illustrates a 15-second commercial:

> **(Definition)** Mary, if you have a minute, I'd like to tell you about a new, important service we have available to our patients. It's called pharmaceutical care.
>
> We decided to begin offering this service because we're finding that some patients have bad reactions to the combination of medications they're taking—prescription and nonprescription. Or, they aren't taking their medications correctly. Did you know that 10%-25% of hospitalizations are from drug-related problems and up to 50% of patients don't take their medicine correctly?
>
> **(Benefits)** I want to be sure our patients get the best possible results from the medications they take, and that's why we're now offering pharmaceutical care. You can schedule an appointment for the evaluation, or ...
>
> **(Price)** The cost of this new service is....

INITIATING A SALE

Although most pharmacists do not see themselves as salespersons, to be successful they must be comfortable talking about pharmaceutical care. Pharmacists do not need to use aggressive sales techniques, but should simply convey the value of their services to their patients. Discussing the features, benefits, and price of pharmaceutical care is key to the success of customer acceptance and buy-in. It is through this conversation that pharmacists will uncover patient needs for pharmaceutical care services.

The pharmacist's first priority is to meet the patient's need. By having a thorough understanding of individual patients' needs, the pharmacist can determine what services and benefits would be of greatest value to them personally. The pharmacist can then connect patient concerns with the benefits of pharmaceutical care. The six-step process for "pitching a sale" outlined in the box on page 143 illustrates this further.

There are numerous opportunities for a pharmacist to identify patients' needs and present the pharmaceutical care services to fit those needs. For example, if a pharmacy offers a disease state management service, potential patients may be identified when they present a new prescription for a medication to treat that specific disease. A quick one-page assessment tool to check patients' understanding and satisfaction with their drug therapy can be used to find patients who need pharmaceutical care. During prospective drug utilization reviews and patient counseling, pharmacists often pinpoint patients who are not compliant or are not achieving the desired outcomes from their therapy. Having a service such

---

SIX-STEP PROCESS FOR PITCHING A SALE

1. **Respond to patient's needs first.** The pharmacist's first priority is to meet the patient's needs. Once the pharmacist has addressed the immediate needs, a transition to the discussion of the pharmaceutical care service can occur.

2. **Make the connection.** Use the conversation with the patient to gather clues to help determine which benefits of pharmaceutical care will be of greatest value to him or her. Then, link the patient's concerns with the solutions that pharmaceutical care offers.

3. **Present services.** Using the link between patient concerns and pharmaceutical care benefits, explain the services offered.

4. **Present price.** After the service and its features and benefits have been fully explained, present the price and package options available and recommend the specific package that seems most appropriate for that patient.

5. **Overcome objections.** Listen carefully to get an indication of what response to expect. If an objection is given, it means the patient is listening but has not been sold on the service. Expect rejection, but don't give up. Research has proven that most people have to hear a marketing message repeated seven to nine times before they are willing to buy.

6. **Ask for the business.** After presenting the services and overcoming objections, it is important that the pharmacist ask the question that confirms agreement. The following are examples of closing and asking for the business:

"Can I set up an appointment for you?" This is the **direct close** and calls for a yes/no decision.

"Would you prefer to set up an appointment today, or would another day work better with your schedule?" The **alternative close** offers options, either of which is a decision to buy.

"I'll need to know about all the medications you're taking now—both prescription and nonprescription— so that I can form a clear picture of your overall medication use." The **assumptive close** is usually an "order-taking" question that follows a patient's decision to buy—the pharmacist "assumes" the sale in this case and continues the steps that have been laid out to the patient for providing pharmaceutical care.

as a general pharmaceutical care program that includes compliance counseling, drug therapy review and evaluation, and the development of a personalized care plan may be of interest to patients having difficulty with their medications.

A change in a patient's physical condition is an opportunity for the pharmacist to offer a disease state management program or a comprehensive review of medications. Perhaps the patient has just been released from the hospital after being treated for disease complications. This may be the best time to offer pharmaceutical care since the need for such services is fresh in the patient's mind.

When discussing the patient's needs concerning nonprescription pharmacotherapy, the pharmacist may uncover an untreated condition or a condition being treated inappropriately. Although receiving reimbursement for these consultations is difficult, such a situation presents an opportunity for pharmacists to enroll patients in pharmaceutical care programs. It is important for pharmacists to use consultations to help promote their services. Looking for opportunities and being ready to offer services that patients need is invaluable. Only by asking will the pharmacist find out if the patient is willing to buy these services.

HANDLING OBJECTIONS

No review of personal selling skills would be complete without discussing how to handle objections. Inevitably, pharmacists will hear objections when attempting to sell a pharmaceutical care service. Objections must be kept in perspective, as they are simply the patient's way of stating what additional information is needed to make a buying decision. An effective model for overcoming objections has the following three steps:

1. **Acknowledge** the objection. Be sure the patient knows the objections were heard. This does not have to be a long, extended response. One of the most effective acknowledgments is simply to say, "I understand how you might feel that way."

2. **Probe** to gain additional information so that responses will be as accurate as possible. Use courteous questioning to find out more about the patient's unique situation so the most valuable features and benefits of pharmaceutical care will be presented.

3. **Respond** to the objection by providing information useful to the patient's decision-making process. This is the time to further define or restate the features and benefits that best resolve the patient's problem and reluctance to buy the service.

PROMOTING PHARMACEUTICAL CARE

Promoting pharmaceutical care services is an essential component of an effective marketing strategy. Pharmacists may assume that by increasing their advertising budget, their promotional strategy is complete, but

OVERCOMING OBJECTIONS TO THE SALE: SOME EXAMPLES

Objection	**"I don't have the time."**
Acknowledge	I know you're really busy.
Probe	Did you know that pharmaceutical care can work out to be a time-saver by keeping you healthy?
Respond	10% to 25% of hospitalizations are a result of problems with medications. And, nearly 50% of prescriptions are taken incorrectly. We think pharmaceutical care will help our patients avoid these problems, which can be a real time saver.
Objection	**"I really don't take a lot of medicine."**
Acknowledge	I know what you mean. It's really a good feeling not to require lots of daily medication and pharmaceutical care can help to keep you healthy.
Probe	Did you know that even nonprescription medications like aspirin, ibuprofen, vitamins, or some of the new heartburn medications can have serious effects on your health if they are taken the wrong way?
Respond	Our pharmaceutical care evaluation gives patients important information that helps ensure the best possible results from medications, and also help them avoid problems. Either way, it's personal information that helps them make better decisions about their own care.
Objection	**"Sounds good, but it seems pretty expensive."**
Acknowledge	I know what you mean. Health care is expensive.
Probe	Have you thought about the cost of the time you spend not recovering as rapidly as you'd like because your medications aren't working as effectively as they could?
Respond	Pharmaceutical care helps you save money by eliminating the cost of physician visits you may have to make if your medications don't work properly. Also, there are several ways to purchase this service...

advertising is just one marketing tool. Pharmacists must look at additional promotional ideas if they are to achieve the personal, professional, and financial success of their practices. Other types of promotional activities are direct mail, publicity, and sales aids. Not only is it important to establish promotional activities for pharmaceutical care services, but also to measure the outcomes and success of each effort. It's the only way to know whether a particular strategy is worthwhile or ineffective.

DIRECT MAIL

Direct mail employs the same format as other marketing techniques, including a review of the product's features and benefits, and can be a very cost-effective promotional tool. When using direct mail, pharmacists should first develop a mailing list and tailor the messages in the mailing to fit the target market.

Keep in mind that writing direct mail copy that brings results is not necessarily easy. Bookstores and libraries carry how-to books on the subject. It's also helpful to look at direct mail pieces already in circulation and evaluate them critically for their characteristics and strengths.

Using the pharmacy's patient database from the computer dispensing system may be the most cost- and time-efficient way to identify potential targets for direct mail. Mailing lists of community members with specific interests (such as diabetes or asthma support groups) are also sometimes available for a price through marketing consultants.

GUIDELINES FOR CREATING DIRECT MAIL PIECES

- Write short paragraphs and simple sentences.
- Focus on the reader and use the word "you."
- Avoid medical jargon.
- Use features and benefits to organize the letter.
- More than one piece of material in a single envelope builds readership. A brochure can be included with the mailing to enhance customer understanding of the service.
- Direct mail experts say that two-page letters tend to bring better results than one page.
- Make sure the letter is at the appropriate reading level.
- Always use a P.S.—it increases readership. (In fact, many people read the P.S. first.)

PUBLICITY

Publicity is a promotional technique that encompasses a number of strategies to target special groups, including making presentations and holding special events. One approach to publicity is presenting oneself to the media as an expert information source. If newspaper, radio, and television reporters realize that a pharmacist is a credible source or interviewee, they will tend to call fairly often for answers to health-related questions. This increases the pharmacist's visibility and may offer opportunities to spotlight particular pharmaceutical care services.

Opinion editorials, news releases, and press releases are additional ways to get the word out about a pharmaceutical care practice. This is usually free publicity and can be a very effective means of marketing. Sending out a news release to the media may not lead directly to a story, but reporters may call to follow up for stories on related topics.

Another way to get the message to patients is to conduct educational seminars or presentations to community groups about pharmaceutical care. Many presentation kits on a number of topics are already available for pharmacists and other health care providers. Presenting the concept of pharmaceutical care "in person" increases the pharmacist's visibility and allows the audience to absorb the message more fully. When looking for presentation opportunities, pharmacists should consider local service groups, church groups, banks, and other business groups—especially those that sponsor activities for people age 50 and over.

> ## SPECIAL EVENTS TO PROMOTE PHARMACEUTICAL CARE
>
> • Appear on radio or television talk shows.
> • Sponsor an entry in a special event.
> • Distribute an article about pharmaceutical care at a health fair or convention.
> • Sponsor a booth or display at a health fair or convention.

Pharmacists can hold or participate in special events to augment the overall marketing strategy. A goal when participating in others' events, such as health fairs, is to gain some recognition for the pharmacy's pharmaceutical care practice. Many pharmacists successfully create their own events, as well—for example, tying a pharmaceutical care smoking cessation program to a special health promotion like the "Great American Smoke-Out." Other events that have proven to be successful include hosting luncheons or brown bag events, staging panel discussions on prescription and nonprescription medications, demonstrating products, and sponsoring open houses. These types of events allow potential patients and local health professionals to see the pharmacist's redesigned pharmacy and learn more about the new service being offered.

SALES PROMOTIONS

Sales promotions include all efforts and materials created to enhance the pharmacist's sales efforts, such as brochures to display on counters or place in patient bags at the point of purchase. With the advent of color printers and photocopiers, professional-looking brochures describing the new pharmaceutical care services are fairly inexpensive to produce. Brochures typically reach current pharmacy patients most effectively. If the pharmacist wishes to reach others in the community with the brochure, a direct mailing may be an option. Other types of sales promotions that are useful include posters, table tents, bag stuffers, coupons, and advertising specialty items.

ADVERTISING

Advertising can be defined as efforts for which pharmacists pay to have messages delivered to target audiences. For advertising to be successful it needs to:

- Be consistent;
- Have a single, clear message;
- Inform, educate, attract, and move the target market into action;
- Be able to break through the "clutter" of messages bombarding consumers daily.

Which media to use for advertising depends on the message that the pharmacist wants to promote, the service being promoted, the target audience, and the budget. Typical advertising choices include print, radio, television, and outdoor advertising.

Radio allows the pharmacist to communicate one-on-one with the consumer. Outdoor advertising, such as billboards, hits a broad target on a regular, consistent basis. Television reaches a comprehensive population base. Newspapers attract a large general readership, yet allow pharmacists to target a population by selecting a specific section of the newspaper for advertising. A new marketing media has developed with the use of home pages on the World Wide Web. Pharmacists need to find the advertising programming that reaches their target market and fits their budget.

PLANNING PROMOTIONAL EVENTS

- Send out invitations and press releases in time for people to make plans. Ask for RSVPs or make follow-up calls.

- Have staff coordinate the various components.

- Let someone else handle the details on the day of the event so the pharmacist can meet and greet the guests.

- Provide a simple item for guests to take with them to remind them of the pharmacy's services.

- Don't try to make one event fit all audiences or stakeholders; instead, schedule different events for different groups.

Radio stations and newspapers will often design ads for their customers at no additional cost. The pharmacist may need to sign a contract specifying a dollar commitment for air time or newspaper space. Alternatively, pharmacists can hire an advertising agency, which may be more creative, but also more expensive. Regardless of the media chosen, it is important to measure the results of advertising efforts to determine each campaign's effectiveness.

PROMOTING BY DOING

It is important to note that the best promotion will come from the actual care provided by pharmacists to patients. Pharmaceutical care is an abstract concept that must be defined—including features and benefits—

to the target audience, but the most effective way to define pharmaceutical care to a patient is to provide it. A satisfied patient becomes the pharmacist's best and least expensive promoter of pharmaceutical care by sharing good experiences with others.

Pharmacists should be cautious about promoting a service that is not quite ready for delivery. Patients who expect one thing but receive another are likely to become frustrated, angry, and dissatisfied. It is essential that pharmaceutical care services be fully developed and prepared for delivery before any full-fledged marketing begins.

TARGETING STAKEHOLDER GROUPS

Promote the new pharmaceutical care service to key people in each of the stakeholder groups, including innovative patients, area physicians, and local employers. Informing people in the community is critical to the success of the pharmacist's practice. Word of mouth and endorsement by influential people in the community helps market the service and build business. These contacts are extremely valuable and important in any marketing strategy. Pharmacists should try to accomplish three goals with each letter, call, or meeting with key contacts:

- Introducing the new service by describing its features and benefits,

- Persuading contacts that the service is valuable,

- Eliciting the contact's support and help.

Physicians are often most receptive to pharmaceutical care when it is explained to them in person. Setting up appointments and explaining the common goal of patient care is an excellent way to begin cooperative relationships with local prescribers. This should be done before any marketing to the public to ensure that physicians are informed and can address questions they may receive from patients about the service.

IMPLEMENTING THE MARKETING STRATEGY

To bring all the individual components together, pharmacists need to create an action plan that complements the marketing plan. As they develop both selling skills and a marketing strategy, pharmacists must address their own objections and personal barriers. Marketing materials is something new for most pharmacists and asking patients and third party payers to pay for cognitive services is not always easy or comfortable.

The action plan must have a timeline and include a realistic budget for promotion—which should be established as part of normal operating expenses. The marketing action plan and timeline, used together, help guide the pharmacist and ensure specific goals are met. Measuring the outcomes of various marketing materials is important for planning future strategies, as noted earlier, but also, when pharmacists see positive movement toward their marketing goals it gives them more confidence to continue.

Conclusion

In the past, pharmacists did not need to market their services, but today it is no longer enough to provide a service and expect people to want it. Identifying the patient's needs, describing the service, discussing the features and benefits, and creating a value for the service are essential components of marketing. Pharmacists must also convey the message that pharmaceutical care is a new type of practice and is extremely valuable to all stakeholders. A successful marketing plan needs extensive attention and ongoing effort.

Because the financial success of pharmaceutical services will depend on reaching, serving, and retaining paying patients, learning how to market pharmaceutical care services should be a priority.

> ### Action Plan to Market Pharmaceutical Care
>
> • Develop a budget.
> • Describe the goal of the marketing effort (the goal).
> • Determine how the pharmacist will achieve the goal (the objective).
> • Identify and describe the target markets (customers and stakeholders).
> • Define key messages.
> • Describe the strategies and tactics to be used.
> • Develop the materials needed to reach the goal.
> • Identify staff members responsible for carrying out the various components of the marketing strategy.

References

1. Shepherd MD. Defining and marketing value added services. *Am Pharm.* 1995;NS35:46-53.

2. Schwartz A, Sogol E. Part 2: Developing a marketing plan. *Drug Topics.* 1987;6:69-75.

3. Smith M. *Pharmaceutical Marketing: Strategy and Cases.* Binghamton, NY: Pharmaceutical Products Press; 1991.

4. Berkowitz E. *Essentials of Healthcare Marketing.* Gaithersburg, MD: Aspen Publishers; 1996.

5. Cooper PD. *Healthcare Marketing.* Gaithersburg, MD: Aspen Publishers; 1994.

6. Kotler P, Armstrong G. *Principles of Marketing.* Upper Saddle River, NJ: Prentice Hall Inc; 1996.

7. Kotler P. *Marketing Management.* Upper Saddle River, NJ: Prentice Hall Inc; 1997.

8. Rogers EM. *Diffusion of Innovations.* New York: New York Press; 1983.

Chapter 10

◆

Reimbursement

For many pharmacists, obtaining reimbursement for pharmaceutical care services is one of the most challenging aspects of implementing pharmaceutical care. One primary obstacle is the limited recognition by patients and payers of pharmaceutical care and its value to the health care system. Pharmacists must engage a strong marketing initiative to change the perceptions and expectations of patients and third party payers about this valuable new service and pharmacists' ability to deliver it.

Another obstacle relates to pharmacists' attitudes in requesting compensation for their knowledge and expertise. Most pharmacists express uneasiness with the role of asking for payment and are concerned about driving patients away. Also, they find it challenging to establish an appropriate pricing methodology and fee for a service that is both new and unique. Procrastination is a factor, as well. Too many pharmacists use the excuse that they will provide pharmaceutical care when they can consistently receive payment for it. Payers respond that they will begin paying for pharmaceutical care once it is consistently delivered and shown to be valuable. To end this stand-off, pharmacists must take charge and begin billing both patients and payers for their new service. Pharmacists also need to track patient outcomes related to drug therapy to demonstrate the value of these services. Only then can they expect to receive reimbursement.

DEFINING THE SERVICE

An important first step in gaining reimbursement for pharmaceutical care is defining the billable services that will be offered. Options may include comprehensive pharmaceutical care and drug regimen reviews, patient education services, health awareness sessions, disease state management services, nonprescription pharmacotherapy consultations, or ancillary services such as immunizations or cholesterol monitoring. Once the service is defined, a pricing methodology and fee must be determined.

When defining the billable pharmaceutical care service, it is very important to distinguish it from traditional pharmacy practice. The federal Omnibus Budget Reconciliation Act of 1990 (OBRA '90) requires pharmacists to maintain patient records, provide prospective drug reviews, and provide patient counseling. Although these tasks are all part of pharmaceutical care, when provided alone they do not represent the ongoing drug therapy management and monitoring that occurs with pharmaceutical care. A pharmaceutical care service also involves regular follow up, goal setting, and outcome measurement and attainment.

The services mandated by OBRA '90 should be considered episodic care, equivalent to a snapshot of patients' drug therapy at the moment they receive a prescription. Pharmaceutical care is continual care that provides an in-depth story of the patient's drug therapy, the patient's health, and the pharmacist's interventions to positively affect the patient's outcome over time.[1] The extensive, patient-focused education of pharmaceutical care is very different from OBRA's basic prescription-driven patient counseling, which is limited to how a specific medication should be used. Also, the comprehensive, in-depth patient history and drug therapy review that is conducted in a pharmaceutical care service is much more thorough than the prospective drug review of a patient's prescription medication list that is required by OBRA '90.

CHANGING PHARMACIST ATTITUDES

Pharmaceutical care is the new standard of practice being embraced by many community pharmacists today. Because pharmaceutical care requires a substantial amount of time and resources, pharmacists should expect to be reimbursed for these services. Unfortunately, this is not consistently happening. No other health professional would be expected to provide such services without reimbursement. However, only a limited number of pharmacists are attempting to charge or submit claims for pharmaceutical care.

Billing patients and third party payers for drug therapy management services is a way to help foster awareness and change expectations about the value of pharmaceutical care. Unless pharmacists are willing to set a fee for these services and begin charging for them, patients and payers will never grasp their value or spend money for them. Stated more bluntly, if pharmacists do not charge for their services they cannot expect to get paid for them.

Some third party payers may not understand this difference between traditional pharmacy practice and pharmaceutical care. They may believe that their basic dispensing fee compensates pharmacists for pharmaceutical care services. An easy example to disprove this belief is when pharmaceutical care results in cancellation of a prescription, and no dispensing fee is paid. Thus, the pharmaceutical care that the pharmacist provides is not recognized by payment, and the pharmacist loses a prescription dispensing fee from the canceled prescription. Also, some patients may ask why they need to pay for a service that has—they believe—been provided free of charge in the past. Thus, a clear distinction between the basic pharmacy service as required by OBRA and the advanced service of pharmaceutical care must be made if efforts to receive reimbursement from both payers and patients are to be successful.

ESTABLISHING A PRICING METHODOLOGY AND FEE

After determining the type of pharmaceutical care services that will be offered, the pharmacist must identify the appropriate pricing methodology and fee. Of the several different pricing methodologies that may be used, the most common are fee-for-service; resource-based, relative value scale (RBRVS); capitation; and cost-savings based pricing systems.

FEE-FOR-SERVICE

Fee-for-service is the "old-fashioned" method of billing for health care: charging a specific rate for a specific service. In the recent era of health care reform, this billing methodology has been criticized because of its inherent incentive to provide more care. Another criticism is that it focuses on payment for actions of the provider, not on fulfilling patient needs.

Managed care is moving to a capitation payment methodology for physicians, as a risk-sharing incentive to limit unnecessary services and hold down costs. Because pharmacists have limited information on the costs of providing pharmaceutical care, an appropriate capitation fee is difficult to determine. Therefore, a fee-for-service approach makes sense when pharmaceutical care is initially being offered. As pharmacists gain more information and knowledge about the financial aspects of providing pharmaceutical care, capitated payment systems may become more prevalent.

Before starting to offer pharmaceutical care, it is critical to develop a pricing methodology and establish fees for each service.

An example of fee-for-service billing is charging a flat hourly rate, so that the fee is based on the time involved. The hourly rate that the pharmacist sets must cover all costs associated with the care provided. Because many of these services are new, however, it may be difficult to accurately estimate their cost. Another possible drawback of an hourly pricing system is that it may motivate the patient to keep the service as brief as possible, thus interfering with the pharmacist's ability to conduct an adequate interview. If an hourly fee system is set, it must be structured to accommodate pharmacists' increased efficiency over time as they become more adept at providing pharmaceutical care.

Other examples of fee-for-service payment methods include a fee established for specific interventions or a fee paid only if a change in therapy or positive outcome occurs. The fee-for-service system was used in the Health Care Financing Administration (HCFA) demonstration project conducted from 1992 to 1996 with the Washington State Medicaid program to pay for cognitive services. Pharmacists were paid $4 for patient interventions of less than six minutes and $6 for those greater than six minutes. Over 20,000 interventions were documented during the 18-month study period. The estimated savings in drug costs was $16 per intervention. After the research project was completed, the Medicaid program opted to continue this payment system.[2]

RESOURCE-BASED, RELATIVE-VALUE SCALE

In the resource-based, relative-value scale pricing methodology, the payment amount is directly related to the level of service provided to the patient. In other words, services are priced according to the amount of time and resources that the patient's care requires. For instance, an asthma patient may need a lengthy data collection session, a complex treatment plan, and regular objective monitoring by the pharmacist, whereas a patient with strep throat may need only a short consultation and one follow-up phone call. In this example, the asthma patient and the strep throat patient would pay different rates due to the differences in the level of pharmaceutical care service provided. Although the RBRVS system is commonly used by physicians, it is not yet well accepted in pharmacy. Because of its complexities and lack of validation for pharmacy, this method may not be easily implemented by pharmacists or readily accepted initially by third party payers.

A pharmacy demonstration project being conducted by Wellmark Blue Cross Blue Shield with several Iowa pharmacies is testing the use of the RBRVS payment system for cognitive services.[3] The demonstration project provides payment, ranging from $14 to $105 per patient each quarter, using the RBRVS payment methodology. Payment for patients with more complex cases, for whom the pharmacists resolve multiple drug therapy problems, is at the higher end of the range, whereas payment for patients who simply need ongoing monitoring but have limited or no drug therapy problems is at the lower end. Unlike with capitation, no payment is made if the patient is not seen and evaluated during that quarter. If multiple patient evaluations are held in one quarter, the quarterly payment is adjusted to a cumulative quarterly amount based on the total number of drug therapy problems identified and resolved for that patient. The project involves 42 Iowa pharmacies and 1,500 patients with asthma, hypertension, diabetes, and ischemic heart disease. Preliminary data show that pharmacists have filed numerous claims for resolving drug therapy problems. In the first few months, quarterly payments to the pharmacies enrolled in the project averaged $590 and ranged from $32 to $1,988.

CAPITATION

The capitation pricing methodology refers to service provided for a fixed fee, usually per patient, per month. The capitation system is particularly appealing to the payer or patient because cost is predetermined at a monthly rate. However, this leaves the provider at risk to keep costs for the capitated patient population below the total monthly capitated amount received for the group. It may be difficult for pharmacists to establish the appropriate capitation figure without historical data on the amount of time spent in patient consultations, and the amount of reimbursement needed to remain profitable. Drug product costs should not be included in the capitated payment unless the pharmacist and prescriber are both at risk for drug product costs and thus have an incentive to keep them low. If the prescriber is not at risk, the pharmacist has limited control over product selection and resulting product costs. Pricing for pharmaceutical care in capitated contracts should reflect these considerations.

Physicians who are involved in contracts for capitated payments for their medical services may be a source of referrals and revenue. A pharmacist can subcontract with physicians to provide time-consuming drug therapy management, thereby allowing physicians to focus the limited time allowed by the capitation rate to other health care needs. An excellent example is pharmacist-managed anticoagulation therapy, which takes an extensive amount of time in educating the patient and numerous patient visits to monitor and stabilize the correct dosage. In this scenario, pharmacists could contract out their drug therapy management services to physicians and establish a set fee per patient. (Keep in mind that pharmacists who subcontract to provide such services must find out from each third party payer the specific rules they must comply with and documentation they must submit with claims. Medicaid, Medicare, and commercial insurance providers may have different requirements for nonphysician providers.)

COST-SAVINGS SYSTEMS

Another pricing methodology relates the fee for pharmaceutical care service to the amount of savings resulting from the pharmacist's intervention. For example, a pharmacist may charge 25% of the annual cost savings achieved from working with the patient and prescribers to cancel an unnecessary chronic medication. This model could yield significant cost savings to the insurer, and it benefits the patient, as well. However, it may be difficult to estimate accurate cost savings for such things as avoiding hospitalization. In addition, not all pharmaceutical care interventions result in cost savings. Compliance monitoring, for example, may actually result in an increased expense for medications. A drawback of this method is that it leaves the pharmacist open to accusations of subjectivity.

In a similar cost-savings pricing approach, pharmacists may work with a payer to share direct pharmacy and medical cost savings achieved for a patient population over time. If the patient population is too small, however, expensive acute health events over which the pharmacist has no control—such as surgery—can skew the results negatively, even though cost savings were achieved with all the other patients. Another disadvantage of this approach is that long-term medical cost avoidance accomplished through preventative health measures is difficult to measure and determine accurately. If this pricing methodology is attempted, the cost data need to be carefully evaluated and fees for acute health care events that inflate costs must be deleted to accurately reflect the pharmacist's impact.

SETTING FEES

Once a pricing methodology has been selected, a fee level must be established. The prices set for pharmaceutical care should take into account the pharmacist's evaluation of the service, the nature of the local market and competition, and the pricing schedule that the market will sustain.

Determining the appropriate fee involves some basic considerations. First, the pharmacist must calculate the actual cost of doing business and determine a reasonable profit. Factors to consider include the pharmacist's salary, benefits, clerical support, and overhead necessary to provide the pharmaceutical care service. Obviously, the fee must be established at a level that will sustain the business practice. This will establish a floor on price. Demand for the service and competition from other providers will determine the ceiling price.

Pharmacists should assess what similar health care providers in the geographic area are charging. Finding out what other professionals, such as the local attorney or financial consultant, are charging for their consulting services may also be helpful. Due to antitrust laws that prohibit sharing of price information among suppliers, it is inappropriate to conduct a fee survey. However, consultants or service firms may have fee information available for sale. Pharmaceutical care services must be priced to fit the community and be competitive with similar services.

Pharmacists need to be realistic in projecting how quickly they can expect to generate revenue. As the service develops and consumer acceptance expands, the revenue generated from pharmaceutical care will increase. Unfortunately, until there is universal understanding and acceptance from patients, employers, and third party payers, pharmacists must invest time and money during the transitional period while getting a low return on investment. For this reason, the pharmacy must be financially stable when pharmaceutical care is implemented so that the economic viability of the business can be maintained during the initial investment period.

Pharmacists may wish to consider establishing a package price that supports their method of delivering a service. For example, a hypertension management program package price may include regular appointments with the pharmacist, routine blood pressure checks, medication compliance packaging, and an annual summary report for the patient and physician. Instead of being essentially "a la carte" pricing, this strategy reflects the group of services as a unit. Package pricing can also be applied to varying levels of services, similar to the bronze, silver, and gold memberships at a health club. The pharmacist should always take the initiative to recommend the appropriate service level for an individual patient. An example of a package pricing grid is shown in Table 1.

The pricing strategy that pharmacists develop should reflect differential pricing for different situations. It is important to remember that few consumers base their buying decisions on price alone. Whatever approach pharmacists adopt for pricing, they should be sure to give it adequate time to work and not change strategies too quickly.

Some pharmacists make the erroneous decision to begin offering pharmaceutical care without having a pricing method in place. When just beginning to learn how to deliver pharmaceutical care, pharmacists may experience feelings of guilt about charging for a service they aren't "good at" yet. Keep in mind that, even though the pharmaceutical care service may not initially be provided quickly and smoothly, it has the same result of identifying and resolving drug therapy problems. If no fees are charged initially, when the pharmacist begins to ask patients for reimbursement there may be extreme resistance and resentment from those patients who previously received the service for free. It is imperative that pharmacists charge for delivering the pharmaceutical care services they develop. To not do so lessens the value of the service and fails to create the positive image needed to change patient and payer perceptions and expectations. Therefore, it is important to have a fee schedule established before offering the service.

SUPPLEMENTARY STRATEGIES

In addition to establishing an appropriate price, some pharmacists have successfully used the "sampling" technique to market their pharmaceutical care services—providing coupons for free evaluations or reduced-price trials. Another approach some pharmacists have tried is having specific patients serve as partners in developing their service by offering it at a discount in exchange for feedback and advice on its improvement. Use of either of these strategies should be limited and discretionary due to the negative perceptions of value that may be created. Also, follow-up tactics must be employed for converting these patients to longer-term "paying" status.

SUBMITTING CLAIMS

Initially, the primary source of payment for pharmaceutical care is the patient. Cultivating a base of cash-paying patients creates a sense

TABLE 1. SAMPLE PRICING/PACKAGING GRID

Plan Type	Includes	Cost
Fee Per Visit	• One-time individual initial evaluation • Analysis communicated to others on health care team	$
Fee Per Multiple Visit	• One individual initial evaluation and two follow-up consultations • Analysis communicated to others on health care team	$$
Annual Membership, Individual	• One individual evaluation and up to three additional consultations per year • Analysis communicated to others on health care team • Reminder notifications	$$$
Annual Membership, Family	• Individual initial evaluations and up to three additional consultations for two adults and up to two children during coverage period • Analysis communicated to others on health care team • Reminder notifications	$$$$

in patients' minds that pharmaceutical care is a valuable service. Unfortunately, pharmacists often overlook the patient as a payer, simply because payments from third parties represent the majority of their revenue. A sign describing the pharmaceutical care products available and their prices should be posted where patients can easily see it. This signage should be supplemented with additional marketing strategies.

Patients interested in the pharmaceutical care service may be able to receive partial or total reimbursement through an insurance plan. Also, the pharmacist can ask for assignment of benefits from the insurance plan (see box on page 159). In the long term, patient demand for pharmaceutical care will help foster payment by third party payers. Although pharmaceutical care has not gained widespread acceptance at this point, awareness of it is growing, and claims are beginning to receive more attention and acceptance by third party payers.

Third party payers usually have several basic concerns when asked to consider payment for pharmaceutical care. Pharmacists must begin by describing pharmaceutical care, its value to patients, and its impact on health care costs. Solid research reports that support these benefits should be supplied. Issues regarding the pharmacist's qualifications or ability to provide this service may arise; payers want to be assured that pharmacists can and will perform to practice standards. In the future, there may be a need to develop credentialing or certification procedures for this purpose.

When pharmacists communicate with third party payers, it is important to identify the appropriate contact person. This should be someone in the medical claims department, not the pharmacy claims division. Drug benefit budgets focus on prescription costs and typically account for around 7% of total health care expenditures. Thus, a bill for cognitive services applied to the pharmacy benefit budget would need to be directly associated with drug cost savings. The budget for medical services, on the other hand, makes up 93% of the health care pie. Due to the potential impact of pharmaceutical care on medical expenses, it is more appropriate to direct claims for pharmaceutical care reimbursement to the medical services budget. It is important to clarify that it is not a drug product claim and that the payment being requested is for a health care service.

REQUESTING ASSIGNMENT

Some pharmacies request assignment of benefits from their patients in an attempt to be more successful at getting reimbursed from third party plans. Assignment of benefits is a statement specifying that the beneficiary will allow the insurer to make payment directly to the health care provider. By authorizing the insurance company to pay the health care provider, the patient is not responsible for filing the paperwork. Accepting assignment means that the pharmacy cannot bill the patient for the service and agrees to accept the amount paid by the insurer.

Services covered by third party payers vary dramatically according to the patient's contract with the payer and various states' laws. As a general rule, the services must be well documented and medically necessary to be paid. When contacting a third party payer, the pharmacist should verify the patient's coverage, deductible, and co-payment. When billing an insurer for the first time, pharmacists should talk to the provider relations department to get essential information, such as services that are covered, forms and coding systems preferred by the insurer, and confirmation about whether the pharmacy can accept assignment.

Some pharmacists prefer to get insurers to agree in advance to cover services before providing the service. If the third party payer declines reimbursement, then the patients are asked to pay for services. If patients refuse to pay, then the services are not provided. Pharmacists should become familiar with each payer's specific policies and procedures for claims submissions and documentation requirements.

If possible, it is in the pharmacist's best interest to obtain a provider number. In most cases this will make claims collection much easier. Several resources provide help and information regarding provider identification numbers. By becoming a certified Medicare durable medical equipment (DME) supplier, the pharmacy receives a Medicare manual that explains billing procedures using the HCFA 1500 form and describes what services are covered. Medicare DME also has a group of local ombudsmen who can provide an orientation program on billing procedures. The regional Medicare carrier can provide a benefits manual with information about DME and Medicare carriers in each state. Information on obtaining provider numbers for private insurance companies can be found by contacting each insurer's provider relations department for its specific policy and procedures.

When pharmacists communicate with third party payers about pharmaceutical care, the appropriate contact person should be in the medical claims department.

Claim Forms

Currently two forms are used most commonly when billing for pharmaceutical care services. The HCFA 1500 claim form is used to bill medical services to an insurance program and is universally recognized and accepted for physician billing. A number of pharmacists have used this recognized form successfully for pharmaceutical care claims payment. The Pharmacist Care Claim Form (PCCF) was developed by the National Community Pharmacists Association (NCPA) to give pharmacists a tool for documenting and billing for pharmaceutical care. Although the PCCF form allows for a more detailed description of the service provided than the HCFA form does, some third party payers have not yet recognized this form and its use by pharmacists. Both the HCFA 1500 form and the PCCF are generated by most prescription dispensing computer software systems. A good approach is to use the recognized HCFA 1500 form and attach the PCCF. Together, the two forms provide a concise and accurate description of the service provided and enhance pharmacists' possibility of receiving reimbursement.

Coding Systems

To bill for pharmaceutical care services, pharmacists need to be familiar with several coding systems, including the ICD-9-CM, HCPCS Level II, and NCPDP PPS codes. ICD-9-CM is the acronym for the International Classification of Diseases, Ninth Revision, Clinical Modification. ICD-9-CM codes are diagnosis codes used by payers to classify illnesses, injuries, and patient encounters with health care providers. These diagnosis codes are necessary to complete HCFA 1500 claim forms, but are not necessary for the PCCF form.

There are three sections of ICD-9-CM codes:

1. General codes for major illnesses.

2. Codes for external causes of injury and poisoning—also known as E codes. This section contains a table of drugs and chemicals that provides general codes to indicate the drug responsible for an adverse effect or poisoning.

3. Codes for exposure to potential health hazards, vaccination, and aftercare—known as V codes.

Pharmacists should use the first section, general codes for major illnesses, as their primary coding section. ICD-9-CM diagnosis codes must be assigned by a physician and given to the pharmacist. The pharmacist should not assign these codes. If, when filing a claim, the pharmacist assigns a diagnosis code to a patient's condition that does not match the ICD-9-CM code assigned by the physician, the claim will be rejected. This situation may also have severe clinical and legal consequences, such as charges of fraud or practicing outside the pharmacist's scope of practice, since assigning a code could be construed as making a medical diagnosis.

> *After filling out claim forms, check them carefully to be sure they are complete. Missing data is the chief reason for third party payers to reject claims.*

Physician Current Procedural Terminology (CPT) codes were developed by the American Medical Association and are updated and published yearly. CPT codes describe medical services and procedures performed by physicians and other health care providers. Many pharmaceutical care services such as patient education, patient care, and consultations are reported with an evaluation and management (E/M) code from the CPT code list. Examples of CPT E/M codes are shown in Table 2.

E/M coding allows a provider to choose from up to five alternative CPT codes to describe a particular service that was performed. The choice of code is based on the level of service that was performed. Three key components—history, examination, and medical decision making—are combined to determine the level of service, which then indicates the amount of compensation. CPT modifiers are extra digits that can be added to the main service or procedure code to indicate that the standard service or procedure has, in some way, been revised. Expanded focused E/M codes in Table 2 are frequently used by practitioners who are billing for pharmaceutical care services. Other codes that are used, depending on the situation and services provided, include consultation E/M codes (99241-99245); confirmatory consultations (99271-99275); case management codes (99361, 99371-99373); and preventive medicine services

TABLE 2. CPT EVALUATION AND MANAGEMENT (E/M) CODES

Patient Type	Code	Definition	Guidelines	Duration
New	99201	Evaluation and management for a self-limited or minor condition	Requires: • A problem-focused history • A problem-focused exam • Straightforward medical decision making	10 min.
New	99202	Evaluation and management for problem(s) of low to moderate severity	Requires: • An expanded problem-focused history • An expanded problem-focused exam • Straightforward medical decision making	20 min.
New	99203	Evaluation and management for problem(s) of moderate severity	Requires: • A detailed history • A detailed exam • Medical decision making of low complexity	30 min.
New	99204	Evaluation and management for problem(s) of moderate to high severity	Requires: • A comprehensive history • A comprehensive exam • Medical decision making of moderate complexity	45 min.
New	99205	Evaluation and management for problem(s) of moderate to high severity	Requires: • A comprehensive history • A comprehensive exam • Medical decision making of moderate complexity	60 min.
Established	99211	Services provided that may not require the presence of the physician	No requirements. Use this level of service when nursing staff performs a blood pressure check, etc.	5 min.
Established	99212	Evaluation and management for a self-limited or minor condition	Requires at least two of the following: • A problem-focused history • A problem-focused exam • Straightforward medical decision making	10 min.

Patient Type	Code	Definition	Guidelines	Duration
Established	99213	Evaluation and management for problem(s) of low to moderate severity	Requires at least two of the following: • An expanded problem-focused history • An expanded problem-focused exam • Medical decision making of moderate complexity	15 min.
Established	99214	Evaluation and management for problem(s) of moderate to high severity	Requires at least two of the following: • A detailed history • A detailed exam • Medical decision making of moderate complexity	25 min.
Established	99215	Evaluation and management for problem(s) of moderate to high severity	Requires at least two of the following: • A comprehensive history • A comprehensive exam • Medical decision making of high complexity	40 min.

Source: Adapted from Coding and Reimbursement Guide for Pharmacists: ICD-9-CM, CPT, HCPCS Level II, NCPDP Codes, Definitions, and Guidelines. *Reston, VA: St. Anthony Publishing, Inc.; 1997.*

(99381-99397, 99401-99412). Pharmacists should refer to the *Coding and Reimbursement Guide for Pharmacists* produced by St. Anthony Publishing for a complete discussion of CPT codes that may be applicable to pharmacy services.[4]

HCFA's Common Procedure Coding System (HCPCS) Level II codes were developed by Medicare and are commonly referred to as national codes. These codes supplement CPT codes and are used for billing Medicare and Medicaid. Some third party payers have also adopted HCPCS codes. These codes are updated periodically throughout the year and are published annually by HCFA. There are HCPCS codes for non-physician services and medical materials or supplies, such as durable medical equipment, new drugs, and office supplies. Guidelines are available that outline the use of these codes and specify the medications that are covered. Medications that cannot be self administered and that require the use of durable medical equipment or infusion equipment are examples of covered drug products. Others include medications used for chemotherapy, dialysis, organ transplantation, and cancer pain management. Although these codes are not used to bill for pharmaceutical care services, they are used to code for materials and supplies that may be necessary for patients who are receiving pharmaceutical care services.[4]

The National Council for Prescription Drug Programs (NCPDP) Professional Pharmacy Service (PPS) codes were modeled after the CPT system and attempt to more accurately define and describe pharmacy-specific cognitive services. PPS codes consist of three fields, each made up of two-character codes that are combined to create a complete code. PPS codes have been incorporated into the PCCF form and have been used in the pharmaceutical care billing process for the Wisconsin Medicaid drug program. The Wisconsin payment system uses a multitiered dispensing fee that pays $4.69 for basic dispensing and a range of $9.08 to $38.55 for spending up to 60 minutes providing pharmaceutical care to a patient.[5]

PPS CODES

Professional Pharmacy Service (PPS) codes consist of three fields, each made up of two-character codes.

- The first field describes the reason for the service, including:
  - Administrative,
  - Dosing/limits,
  - Drug conflicts,
  - Disease management,
  - Precautionary reasons.
- The second is the action field, which describes the professional or administrative service provided by the pharmacist.
- The third is the result field, which describes how the problem was resolved:
  - Dispensed,
  - Not dispensed,
  - Patient care.
- A code indicating the level of service provided during the encounter may also be given as a fourth field. This code is determined by the complexity of the decision-making process or resources used by the pharmacist, as well as the time required to perform the service.

Before submitting a claim for pharmaceutical care, it is important to proofread it, making sure that every blank is completed and that the information provided is accurate and straightforward. Missing data is the chief cause of claim rejection. The pharmacist may also want to generate a billing invoice, especially if a claim form is not used. The patient's co-pay should be factored in if appropriate. A cover letter with a complete description of services rendered may be included with the claim to explain the contents of the form.

Sometimes, to ensure payment of a claim, a pharmacist may need to obtain a certificate of medical necessity from a physician. Payers may want proof that the services provided are appropriate to the patient's condition. A certificate of medical necessity can be thought of as a prescription order for a pharmaceutical care service. This certificate is completed by the physician and includes the patient's ICD-9-CM diagnosis codes, the pharmaceutical care services that the physician is requesting for the patient, the anticipated duration of service, and the physician's signature. In some cases, where the patient is requesting the service, a certificate of medical necessity may be filled out by the patient. A claim that is accompanied by a certificate of medical necessity may have a better chance of being paid because it communicates that the physician or patient believed the service was necessary. This tactic is somewhat controversial, for though it may help the pharmacist obtain payment for claims, it also poses a danger of tying pharmaceutical care reimbursement only to a physician's order.

Most insurance companies require some co-payment or deductible. The amount or percentage will vary depending on the insurance company and the program. It is important that the pharmacist know the terms of the patient's insurance program in advance. The pharmacist must bill the patient for any co-pay or deductible. If the patient is unable to pay, these fees can be waived, but the pharmacist must make an attempt to collect payment; otherwise, the pharmacist has committed insurance fraud.

Handling a Rejected Claim

If a pharmacist's claim is rejected by a third party payer, the pharmacist can then set up an appointment with the payer's case manager to discuss the claim further. If the case manager also denies the claim, a clinical pharmacist from the medical benefits division of the insurance program should be contacted. At each of these meetings, the pharmacist should be prepared to show evidence that the pharmaceutical care services were medically necessary (certificate of medical necessity), provide documentation of the service from the patient's chart, present any referrals or recommendations made, and indicate what the outcome could have been had the service or intervention not occurred. In the event that the payer still will not accept the claim, the pharmacist may contact the patient's employee benefits manager, who may be willing to speak to the payer on behalf of the employee. If, after exploring all these options, the claim has still not been paid, the pharmacist should seek reimbursement from the patient.

Educating Payers

Educating payers about the value of pharmaceutical care is an effective way to increase reimbursement. Pharmacists should consider forming local task forces and visiting payers as a group to explain the concept and value of pharmaceutical care. When meeting with payers, be prepared to show projected savings and other benefits that will result from coverage. Stress the benefits to the payer's company and to the patient.

It may be beneficial for several pharmacists located in the same geographic area to form a cooperative initiative. This group could pool marketing resources for contacting local physicians, employers, and third party payers to inform them of the services that member pharmacies are providing. Such a group could help to ensure that a common message is conveyed and that a standard of practice is established for pharmaceutical care within a community.

CONCLUSION

Reimbursement is an extremely important issue for the success of pharmaceutical care and the future of the pharmacy profession. Factors that contribute to the success of achieving reimbursement are the pharmacist's confidence in the services provided, having a payment schedule in effect, researching possible payers and cultivating these payers, and submitting the proper forms with the proper codes. Creating positive relationships with other pharmacists, payers, and physicians will also enhance the pharmacist's chances of full reimbursement for pharmaceutical care services. Once the pharmacist helps patients and payers better understand and appreciate the benefits of pharmaceutical care, more and more claims will be paid in full.

REFERENCES

1. Graves M, McDonough R. Making reimbursement a reality in pharmaceutical care. *Iowa Pharmacist.* 1997;51(6):15-21.

2. Christensen DB, Holmes GH, Andrews A, et al. Payment of pharmacists for cognitive services: results of the Washington State C.A.R.E. demonstration project. Medical Assistance Administration Department of Social and Health Services State of Washington, Department of Pharmacy, School of Pharmacy, University of Washington. December 1996.

3. Anon. Wellmark demo project update. *Insights—Official Newsletter of the Iowa Pharmacists Association.* 1997;1(13):8-9.

4. *Coding and Reimbursement Guide for Pharmacists: ICD-9-CM, CPT, HCPCS Level II, NCPDP Codes, Definitions, and Guidelines.* Reston, VA: St. Anthony Publishing, Inc.; 1997.

5. Gillard M, Whitmore S. The Wisconsin Medicaid pharmaceutical care project. *Wisconsin Pharmacist.* May/June 1996:7-14.

Chapter 11

◆

Drug Information Skills for Pharmaceutical Care

BY KEVIN MOORES, PHARM.D.
DIRECTOR, IOWA DRUG INFORMATION NETWORK
THE UNIVERSITY OF IOWA COLLEGE OF PHARMACY

This chapter provides an overview of the drug information skills pharmacists need to practice pharmaceutical care and the processes and philosophy involved in answering drug information questions. As described in Chapter 2, one of the key steps in providing pharmaceutical care is identifying actual or potential drug therapy problems. Once identified, a drug therapy problem may, in essence, be viewed as a drug information question.

To provide pharmaceutical care, pharmacists must obtain, use, and provide patient-specific drug information and must have access to accurate, up-to-date information about medications, diseases, and developments in professional practice. According to guidelines from the American Society of Health-System Pharmacists, "the provision of medication information is among the fundamental professional responsibilities of pharmacists in health systems."[1] These guidelines recommend a systematic approach to providing medication information. They also state that "medication information may be patient specific, as an integral part of pharmaceutical care, or population based, to aid in making decisions and evaluating medication use for groups of patients. The goal of providing carefully evaluated, literature-supported evidence to justify medication-use practices should be to enhance the quality of patient care and improve patient outcomes."

A consensus document developed at a 1991 conference of drug information educators and practitioners held in Albuquerque, New Mexico, emphasizes that as an integral part of pharmaceutical care, pharmacists must use a systematic approach to applying data from published literature to patient care.[2] Most colleges of pharmacy in the United States have adopted the drug information education objectives agreed upon at the conference for use in their curricula. The document also serves as a useful tool for designing drug information skill development programs or continuing education programs for practitioners.

> ## KEY STEPS IN PROVIDING MEDICATION INFORMATION
>
> 1. Assess the medication information needs of patients, families, and health care professionals.
> 2. Conduct interviews and gather data to formulate a specific answerable question related to the patient's care.
> 3. Perform a search for the best available evidence applicable to the question.
> 4. Evaluate the evidence.
> 5. Create a synthesis of the evidence and develop a response or therapeutic plan.
> 6. Communicate the response or recommendation.
> 7. Document recommendations and actions.
> 8. Follow up to evaluate the success of recommendations, the therapeutic response, and the potential need for additional information.

FORMULATING QUESTIONS

Regardless of how the need for drug information is generated—directly by the pharmacist or as a question from another health care provider, the patient, or the patient's family—the process of providing a response is almost always the same. The first step is to formulate a clear, accurate, answerable question. Defining the question, similar to generating a hypothesis for a research study, prepares the information provider for the next step: searching for relevant evidence. A well-organized literature search will typically include all or at least parts of four elements that make up a well-formed clinical question:

1. A description of the patient that details the current problem and all factors that could be relevant to drug therapy decisions (comparable to inclusion/exclusion criteria in high-quality clinical trials);
2. Identification of a potential intervention (e.g., add a new drug, discontinue a drug, change a dose);
3. Possible alternatives to the potential intervention (e.g., an alternative drug, a nondrug therapy, or no therapy);
4. The desired specific outcome (e.g., relieve symptoms of depression, cure an infection, avoid the side effect of drowsiness from medication).

HISTORICAL BACKGROUND FOR THE QUESTION

When pharmacists have finished taking a history in preparation for answering a drug information question, they should have recorded several details (see box on page 170). In the process of formulating the question the pharmacist will classify it two ways—by the requestor (taking into account the person's background, level of understanding, and plans for using the information) and by the information requested (dose, drug interaction, adverse drug reaction, product availability, drug selection, etc.). Classifying the question helps pharmacists formulate an initial hypothesis as they address the question and consider possible solutions, and it helps them focus their answers.

A pharmacist may wish to use a structured data collection form to organize patient history and relevant background information related to a patient-specific drug information request, and to document the information and recommendations provided. A sample form appears at the end of this chapter.

EVIDENCE-BASED HEALTH CARE

The concepts in this chapter are linked to the philosophy of evidence-based health care. Evidence-based health care may be defined as the "conscientious, explicit, and judicious use of current best evidence in making decisions about the care of individual patients."[3]

In practice, evidence-based health care (also referred to as "evidence-based medicine") integrates individual clinical expertise with the best external clinical evidence available from systematic research. Evidence-based health care is often mistaken for, or reduced to, just one of its several components—the critical appraisal of the literature. However, evidence-based health care requires both clinical expertise and an intimate knowledge of a patient's situation, beliefs, priorities, and values. Clinical expertise determines if external evidence may be applied to a patient, and if so, how it should be used in decision-making by the patient and by the health care provider.

The pharmacist must consider the complete context of a question, including the detailed characteristics of the medical condition(s), risk factors of the patient involved, and other important patient-specific details (see Chapter 3). Also, the pharmacist must clearly understand why the question is being asked, who will receive the information, and how the information will be used.

Jumping at the first expressed question is tempting but notoriously inefficient and often leads to errors in decision-making. If a response is met with several new questions, the pharmacist clearly did not address the information needs of the requestor and should improve interview, history-taking, and assessment skills.

DETAILS TO RECORD BEFORE ANSWERING A DRUG INFORMATION QUESTION

- The date and time of the request,
- How the request was received (telephone, fax, e-mail, in person),
- Who is requesting the information,
- The requestor's background (patient, physician, pharmacist, nurse, etc.),
- How to contact the requestor to provide the information and follow-up,
- What information they requested,
- How the information is to be used,
- Why they asked for the information,
- What background is pertinent (patient-specific or other details behind the question),
- The pharmacist's description of the specific answerable question,
- When the information is needed.

Inexperienced practitioners commonly rush through the history-taking process and make assumptions about the patient's situation or why certain information is requested during drug therapy consultations. The person requesting information may leave out important points, assuming that only certain details are relevant. If overlooked in the beginning stages, false assumptions accumulate to become dangerous barriers to clear communication. Examples of general and specific background details to obtain, based on the type of information requested, are provided at the end of this chapter.

In some cases a question may appear very obvious and simple, such as, "What are the available tablet strengths for Serzone?" Without knowing the specific purpose of the question, the pharmacist may make inappropriate assumptions about the requestor's information needs and simply respond with facts about the tablet strengths even though the question may be more involved. For example, a patient may have experienced an adverse reaction. In response, a physician may have decided to reduce the dose of Serzone and is asking the pharmacist about available tablet strengths, to find out if a smaller tablet size is available. This decision may be based on inappropriate assumptions about the cause of the patient's symptoms, the safety and efficacy of various doses of the medication, and the options available to adjust the dose.

A question involving a potential adverse reaction requires detailed information for a proper solution to the actual drug therapy problem. The specifics of the patient's symptoms, the potential causes of the symptoms, and numerous other clinical details are relevant. A patient may be experiencing typical, minor, self-limited side effects that will diminish in a short time, or may be taking other medications that are causing a potentially dangerous interaction. The patient may have a hypersensitivity to the medication, may be having a reaction to another medication entirely, or may possibly be showing symptoms of a new, undiagnosed medical condition. Without knowing the relevant background information, any of these possibilities may go undetected by the pharmacist. Because the proper response to each of these situations may be very different, the pharmacist should always determine why the initial question was asked. Even if the requestor's decision to reduce the dose turns out to be the correct action, it is still possible that the question was not optimally defined and answered.

TACTFUL PROBING

The pharmacist must develop a certain amount of skill and tact to obtain the information needed to address drug therapy questions effectively. Background questions asked by the pharmacist must be appropriate for the circumstances, must be handled efficiently, and must demonstrate competence so as to gain the requestor's confidence.

In the example on the previous page, in which the physician asks about available strengths for Serzone, the pharmacist could not start by asking, "Why do you want to know?" There is no tactful way to ask that specific question. The pharmacist could begin with a phrase like, "Yes, I can get that information for you. Does this question relate to therapy for a specific patient?" If the answer is a simple "Yes," the pharmacist may then ask, "Are they having a problem with their therapy?" The response will help the pharmacist learn enough to ask specific questions and provide accurate, appropriate recommendations.

MORE RESOURCES

Additional information on taking a drug: information history and formulating specific, relevant, answerable questions is available from the following resources:

- Galt KA. *The ASHP Clinical Skills Program Drug Information Module 1: Analyzing and Recording a Drug Information Request.* Bethesda, MD: American Society of Health-System Pharmacists; 1994.— Provides extensive information on determining the needed drug information and collecting patient-specific data. Also details communication skills and interviewing strategies, and includes case examples.

- Sackett DL, Richardson WS, Rosenberg W, Haynes RB. How to ask clinical questions you can answer. In: *Evidence-Based Medicine: How to Practice and Teach EBM.* New York: Churchill Livingstone; 1997: 21-36.

- Kirkwood CF. Modified Systematic Approach to Answering Questions. In: Malone PM, Mosdell KW, Kier KL, Stanovich JE, eds. *Drug Information: A Guide for Pharmacists.* Stamford, CT: Appleton & Lange; 1996: 15-26.

Evidence-based medicine web sites with articles on tailoring clinical questions and other useful tools:

- Centre for Evidence-Based Medicine, Oxford, England: http://cebm.jr2.ox.ac.uk/

- Health Information Research Unit, McMaster University, Hamilton, Ontario: http://hiru.mcmaster.ca/.

Within the time it takes to pull the information up on a computerized drug information reference, or look in a standard text, the pharmacist can ask one or two additional questions to verify assumptions and assess the requestor's need for more information. This way, the response is not delayed if the question is quick and straightforward, but the pharmacist takes the opportunity to see if more detailed information is necessary.

If pharmacists communicate with confidence and show concern that their advice will serve the patient's best interest, their need to know the circumstances of the question will be respected. If pharmacists already have established relationships with health care providers who know the value of their therapeutic knowledge and recommendations, those providers will typically supply appropriate patient background as a matter of course.

SEARCHING FOR INFORMATION

To be effective, health professionals must maintain clinical competence and awareness of the most effective therapies for preventing or treating illness. The skills to efficiently search the literature for the best evidence to support drug therapy decisions are critical to answering complex patient-specific questions. Drug and medical information resources may all be classified into one of three broad categories: primary, secondary, and tertiary literature.

- Primary literature is original biomedical research published as journal articles. It contains the most current and detailed information for determining if conclusions are likely to be applicable to an individual patient. The disadvantages of primary literature are that it can be difficult to locate the needed information, and that experience and skill are needed to properly evaluate and interpret it.

- Secondary literature includes the abstracting and indexing services that organize the millions of articles published in the primary literature. Secondary literature databases used by most pharmacists include Medline (from the National Library of Medicine), International Pharmaceutical Abstracts (from the American Society of Health-System Pharmacists), and the Iowa Drug Information Service (from the University of Iowa College of Pharmacy). Strategies for using secondary resources are detailed on pages 177-178 and 179. Advantages of secondary sources include ease of use and comprehensiveness of the information. A key disadvantage is that the database may contain only abstracts and it may be time-consuming or costly to obtain the full-text article. Many pharmacists need additional training to use secondary sources well. New technology and networks are reducing barriers to accessing and using these powerful databases.

SOME NEW TYPES OF INFORMATION RESOURCES

BEST EVIDENCE

Best Evidence is a CD-ROM database of the journals *ACP Journal Club* and a similar publication, *Evidence-Based Medicine.* *ACP Journal Club* has been published by the American College of Physicians (ACP) since 1991. It uses explicit criteria of clinical importance and methodological standards to select original research articles previously published in other journals. The editors then write an abstract and expert commentary, place the results of the original article in context with previous research, and recommend uses for the information in practice. *Evidence-Based Medicine,* a joint publication from the ACP and the British Medical Journal Publishing Group, includes articles related to family practice, surgery, psychiatry, pediatrics, internal medicine, and obstetrics and gynecology.

To search Best Evidence, a searcher simply types in key words related to the information desired and the program searches the CD-ROM for articles containing those terms. Examples that one might search include peptic ulcer disease and helicobacter pylori, beta-blockers and myocardial infarction, or any number of topics that would involve decision-making for drug therapy. The advantage of using a resource like Best Evidence is that the editors prescreen the content for validity and applicability to practice.

Best Evidence's disadvantages are similar to those of textbooks. The database is not comprehensive, some of the material may be out of date, and users are somewhat dependent on the experts' opinions, although the abstracts do provide more detail on the original study data than will be found in textbooks. More information about Best Evidence can be obtained from this web site: http://www.acponline.org/catalog/cbi/.

COCHRANE LIBRARY

The Cochrane Library is a collection of four databases on one CD-ROM: The Cochrane Database of Systematic Reviews, The York Database of Abstracts of Reviews of Effectiveness, The Cochrane Controlled Trials Register, and The Cochrane Review Methodology Database.

The Cochrane Database of Systematic Reviews is a collection of highly structured reviews of research evidence in specific areas of health care. Data are often combined statistically (by meta-analysis) to increase the power of the findings from multiple studies. Currently this database includes 377 complete reviews on such topics as interventions to assist patients with adherence to drug therapy regimens; analgesic and anti-inflammatory therapy in osteoarthritis; and antibiotic therapy for acute bronchitis.

The Cochrane Controlled Trials Register is a bibliography of controlled trials identified by contributors to the Cochrane Collaboration as part of an international effort to create an unbiased source of data for systematic reviews of the medical literature. Approximately 180,000 articles are referenced in this bibliography.

The Cochrane Review Methodology Database is a bibliography of articles and books on the science of research evaluation and synthesis. It also contains an extensive handbook on conducting critical literature appraisal and how to develop systematic reviews of the best available evidence on health care topics. More information is available about the Cochrane Collaboration and the Cochrane Library from the McMaster University evidence-based medicine web site: http://hiru.mcmaster.ca/cochrane/default.htm.

- Tertiary literature includes review articles, textbooks, compendia, and full-text computerized databases. The advantage of using tertiary resources is that the information has been reviewed and condensed so it is more compact and quicker to study. The key disadvantage is that the information, in even the best texts, is one to three years old the day it is printed. Also, since the information is condensed, the level of detail diminishes, and the reader must rely on the author's opinion for many of the recommendations cited. Verifying the accuracy of information in tertiary resources is often difficult and time-consuming.

CLINICAL PRACTICE GUIDELINES

Clinical practice guidelines and systematic reviews are tertiary resources developed significantly in the last five years. These resources are very helpful for pharmacists looking for authoritative information about the use of medications to treat or prevent disease.

Examples of clinical practice guidelines that every pharmacist should have available are:

- *The Sixth Report of the Joint National Committee on Prevention, Detection, Evaluation, and Treatment of High Blood Pressure*— "JNC VI" from the National Institutes of Health (NIH);
- *The National Asthma Education and Prevention Program Expert Panel Report II: Guidelines for the Diagnosis and Management of Asthma;*
- *The National Cholesterol Education Program* (NCEP);
- *American College of Chest Physicians Consensus Conference on Antithrombotic Therapy;*
- *NIH Consensus Development Panel on Helicobacter pylori in Peptic Ulcer Disease;*
- *American College of Gastroenterology Medical Treatment of Peptic Ulcer Disease;*
- *Depression in Primary Care: Clinical Practice Guideline* from the Agency for Health Care Policy and Research (AHCPR);
- *Guide to Clinical Preventive Services: Report of the U.S. Preventive Services Task Force.*

There are additional guidelines from the AHCPR related to acute pain, chronic pain, benign prostatic hyperplasia, heart failure, angina, and other topics. Many other documents are available from the American Heart Association, the American Diabetes Association, and other organizations. Some of these guidelines are published in the medical literature, some are available from the federal government, some may be purchased from the professional associations that produced them, and many are available at various web sites. The AHCPR is coordinating a national guideline clearinghouse: see http://www.ahcpr.gov.

SEARCH STRATEGIES

The initial strategy for a search depends on the nature of the question and also on the pharmacist's own background knowledge or understanding of available information on a topic. Pharmacists planning to research a topic in which they have a limited background, or that they have not reviewed for some time, should start with a tertiary resource.

> *Clinical practice guidelines are systematically developed statements to help practitioners and patients make decisions about appropriate health care for specific circumstances.*

For example, if the question relates to the safety and efficacy of a new drug, like carvedilol for treating heart failure, the searcher should be familiar with the details of heart failure, such as:

- Presenting symptoms,
- Appropriate methods for evaluating severity of heart failure,
- Natural course of the disease,
- Risk factors for the disease,
- Prognostic indicators,
- Typical response that may be achieved with standard therapy,
- How to monitor response to therapy.

A searcher unfamiliar with these issues will not be prepared to evaluate the evidence retrieved concerning the efficacy and safety of carvedilol compared to other treatments.

One resource useful for this type of background information is a therapeutics textbook, like *Pharmacotherapy: A Pathophysiologic Approach* by Dipiro et al., or a textbook of internal medicine. Another good alternative would be a clinical practice guideline or a systematic review. For example, a clinical practice guideline, *Heart Failure: Evaluation and Care of Patients with Left-Ventricular Systolic Dysfunction,* is available from AHCPR on its web site. A guideline is available from a joint task force of the American College of Cardiology and the American Heart Association, published in *Circulation* (1995;92:2764-84), and an excellent review article by Jay Cohn, MD, one of the most recognized experts in the treatment of heart failure, is in the *New England Journal of Medicine* (1996;335:490-8).

After studying a few of the guidelines or reviews on heart failure, the pharmacist would search for specific studies on the use of carvedilol, preferably randomized controlled trials, and possibly a meta-analysis of trials with carvedilol.

How does one find these references without a drug information center or a medical library close by? One bibliographic database now available "virtually" everywhere is Medline. In June 1997 the National Library of Medicine announced that both PubMed and Internet Grateful Med would be available free on the Internet, greatly simplifying access to Medline for health professionals and the public.

USE OF THE INTERNET

Access to the Internet should be considered a standard feature of every pharmacy practice. A vast amount of information is available via the Internet, which is both a benefit and a serious detriment. A key rule that pharmacists should keep in mind is, trust no one. Other rules include: nobody is in charge, everything changes rapidly and often, and the user must take an organized and measured approach to the Internet to be successful.

The part of the Internet that has gained the most attention in the last few years is the World Wide Web, which allows access to text, graphics, audio, and video. Among components that web users should be familiar with are:

> **TOUR GUIDES TO THE INTERNET**
>
> For further information about the organization of and uses for different components of the Internet, there are several useful tutorial and "tour guide" resources available on the web. One such resource, maintained by the University of Iowa Libraries, is called the Gateway to the Internet and is found at http://www.lib.uiowa.edu/gw/ .

- The browser. A new web user should first learn the features and functions of this software, which connects users to web sites. The most common browsers are Netscape Navigator and Internet Explorer. Each of these programs has help features and Internet sites to provide education on the software.

- Search engines. These are free services that search the web to find information based on key words input by the user. As of this writing, the most common search engines include: AltaVista, Excite, HotBot, Infoseek, Lycos, Webcrawler, and Yahoo. Most users learn to manipulate one or two search engines very well and use them as their primary gateways to information on the Internet. All the search engines listed above have help features and web sites to provide instruction. When using a search engine to find information, always remember the cardinal rule of the Internet: everything changes quickly and often.

- Internet directories. Many subject directories are currently available both in print and on the web, and many more become

SEARCHING MEDLINE

Many different software systems are available for searching Medline and each has advantages and disadvantages for ease of use and ability to perform advanced search functions. A few general principles apply to searching most bibliographic databases, including Medline. Although this overview provides general tips, it would be helpful to find a continuing education course for hands-on practice and instruction from an experienced searcher.

The indexes to these databases are created by using specific controlled vocabularies to describe the information content of the indexed articles. For best results, a pharmacist must use the same vocabulary to search the database. In the case of Medline, the controlled vocabulary is called Medical Subject Headings (MeSH) and contains more than 14,000 terms. An excellent review describes the MeSH vocabulary and is highly recommended reading.[4]

A FEW KEY POINTS:

- MeSH terms come from a hierarchical or tree-branching structure in which specific terms are arranged under more general terms. For example, the drug term fluoxetine is in a tree structure under serotonin uptake inhibitors, which is under neurotransmitter uptake inhibitors, which is under neurotransmitter agents, which after a couple more steps is under chemicals and drugs, the highest level in the tree structures.

- In most cases the specific term is preferred for searching, because the indexers are taught to use the most specific term applicable to the subject.

- When users want to search for an entire category of drugs, they generally choose the category name and use it as an exploded term, which means they simultaneously search both the broad category term and the more specific terms in the tree structure. (If the software permits, it is helpful to view the tree structure when using this method to see what is actually being searched.)

- When dealing with new concepts or new drugs not yet assigned a specific term, searchers may want to use a combination of text word searching and MeSH terms. Text words are words that appear in the title or abstract of an article.

- Truncation may also be used to search for words that begin with a given text string but have variable endings. The symbol to use truncation varies with different software; the most frequent symbol is an asterisk (*). For example, searching bacter* would include bacteria, bacterium, bacteriophage, bacteroides, etc.

- Determining the correct MeSH term for a concept is not always obvious. For example, the MeSH term for congestive heart failure is "heart failure, congestive." Depending on the system, the software may map the terms that have been input to the appropriate MeSH term, or the pharmacist may need to use an online electronic thesaurus to find the correct term.

- The National Library of Medicine publishes a print version of the MeSH terms, which may be used to look up the terms manually.

- A collateral search is another way to

SEARCHING MEDLINE *(CONTINUED)*

identify accepted MeSH terms using text words. A searcher reviews the records retrieved for relevance, studies the MeSH terms used to index a specific article, and re-inputs those terms to find related articles.

- Another useful feature of the MeSH vocabulary is called subheadings: approximately 80 terms that can be applied to the use of the main MeSH terms. For example, a searcher using a drug term may wish to attach subheadings such as therapeutic use, toxicity, adverse effects, poisoning, or pharmacokinetics to that term. By applying the subheadings, searchers can narrow the articles retrieved to those that deal with a specific aspect of a particular drug.

- A powerful feature of computerized database search systems is the ability to combine search terms with the Boolean expressions "and," "or,"

"not." By combining terms with "and," both terms would have to appear in the indexing record for the article to be retrieved. Using "or" would get articles that include either term. Using "not" makes it possible to specifically exclude a subset of articles, such as those dealing with animal studies.

- Searchers may also use a variety of tools called search limits or filters that restrict the results to certain years, to English language, to human data, to selected age groups, and other options depending on the system. In addition, searchers may limit their search to publication types such as randomized controlled trials, meta-analysis, and practice guidelines. Articles may also be found by searching author name, author location, and journal title.

---

available every day. These directories, created by academic institutions, professional associations, and commercial companies, keep up-to-date lists of web site links grouped under categorical headings. By clicking on the link, the browser takes the user to the site automatically. The best way to learn to use directories is to choose a few, experiment with them, and try new sites.

EVALUATING INFORMATION ON THE INTERNET

Evaluating the validity of information on the Internet is difficult since the peer review process that pharmacists are familiar with for published journals is rarely applied there. A key to judging reliability of information from an Internet site is knowing the reputation of the sponsor. Sites from organizations like the American Pharmaceutical Association, the American Society of Health-System Pharmacists, the American Medical Association, the American Diabetes Association, the American Heart Association, and government agencies like the Food and Drug Administration (FDA) are generally more reliable than the average site that ends in ".com."

It would be impossible to provide here a complete review of principles for evaluating information on the Internet, but a few key criteria to consider are:

- Authorship. Who is the author of the information and what are the author's credentials?

- Referencing. Does the author provide credible references to the primary literature to support the conclusions?

- Disclosure. Is there any potential conflict of interest on the part of the author and is information regarding this potential disclosed on the site?

- Currency. What is the date of last revision of the information and how current are the references to the literature?

EVALUATING PRIMARY LITERATURE

Detailing the process of evaluating the primary literature would take far more space than this chapter allows. A key aspect is understanding basic principles for determining internal validity of a study (the "truth" or findings that apply to patients in the study) and external validity (the ability to extrapolate the results to make judgments for patients not actually in the study). The basic design of the trial must be considered carefully. Each of the common major research designs, listed below, has particular

THE IOWA DRUG INFORMATION SERVICE DATABASE

The Iowa Drug Information Service (IDIS) database is designed specifically for retrieving information about the use of drugs to treat, prevent, or diagnose disease in humans. Updated monthly, the IDIS database is created from 200 leading English language pharmacy and medical journals, about one-fourth of which are published outside the United States. Each record in the database includes the article title, author(s), journal source, index terms, and cross reference terms. Similar to Medline, approximately 60% of recent articles include an abstract in the CD-ROM searchable database.

Like Medline, the IDIS database uses a hierarchical drug vocabulary arranged by therapeutic categories. The U.S. Adopted Name (USAN) is the generic drug name used in the database. The main advantage of the IDIS drug vocabulary is that it is kept more up to date and is more complete and specific than the MeSH terms (see page 177).

The disease terminology used in the IDIS database is a modification of ICD-9-CM (defined in Chapter 10). More than 150 descriptor terms are defined in the database to label the specific characteristics of each article entered.

Although the IDIS database is not as comprehensive as Medline, it offers advantages because of the specificity of the database, the specificity of the drug terms and descriptors, the focus on English language articles related to the use of drugs in humans, and the availability of full-text articles. The IDIS database is available on CD-ROM, online, on the Internet, and on microfiche. For more information about this database see the web site: http://www.uiowa.edu/~idis/ .

strengths and weaknesses in terms of internal and external validity, feasibility, costs, time and resource requirements, and ethics.

- Randomized controlled clinical trials. This is the gold standard for evaluating drug therapy and is required by the FDA to prove that a drug is effective and safe;
- Nonrandomized prospective cohort studies;
- Nonrandomized historical case control studies;
- Cross sectional surveys;
- Case series or case reports.

The following is a brief outline of key questions to ask when evaluating a randomized controlled trial:

- Was assignment of patients truly random and was the randomization process effective in concealing assignment?
- Were all patients in the trial accounted for in the results?
- Was the analysis done by the principle of intention to treat?
- Were the patients and the investigators successfully blinded to treatment?
- Were the two groups equal at baseline and were they treated equally other than for the specific study treatment?
- Were the patients representative of the target population or a population similar to those patients seen in practice?
- Were the outcomes measured appropriate, accurate, and sensitive?
- If the results of the study were negative (a difference was not found), was the statistical power of the trial assessed?
- Was the control treatment (a placebo or other active treatment) the appropriate comparison to make?
- Were there violations of the protocol?
- If the effect was statistically significant was it also clinically significant?
- Was the study of adequate duration so that the results are comparable (or at least predictive) to the duration of the treatment as it would be used in practice?

Pharmacists who have not had a formal course in primary literature evaluation may wish to enroll in a continuing education program or a self-study course. The ability to accurately assess published literature will continue to grow in importance as pharmacists expand their roles in drug therapy decision-making and in educating patients and health care providers. A bibliography of resources for evaluating the literature appears on page 184.

FORMULATING A RESPONSE

Assuming that, at this point, the pharmacist has not only formulated a specific, relevant, answerable drug information question but has also systematically searched for the best evidence and evaluated it, the next step is to adjust the response to the informational needs of the requestor.

It is helpful for the pharmacist to summarize the information and recommendations in a brief logical statement. The recommendation should take into consideration patient-specific details collected in the interview and data gathering process. For example, if a patient requires dosage adjustment because of age, reduced renal or hepatic function, or concomitant illness or medications, these factors should be included in the response formulated by the pharmacist.

In very simple cases, such as adjusting a dosage or discontinuing a drug, it may not be necessary to supply specific supporting evidence for the recommendation. If the response is provided to another health care professional, however, the pharmacist should be prepared to explain the reasoning and tell the requestor where supportive information may be found.

> ### CLINICAL TRIALS VS. OUTCOMES STUDIES
>
> There is debate about the overall usefulness of randomized controlled trials (RCTs) for decision-making in clinical practice. Although RCTs provide the highest level of statistical power to determine internal validity in a study, they sometimes suffer in terms of external validity. It can be difficult to extrapolate the results beyond the limits of the patients in the trial because the strict controls used to enhance compliance, monitor patients, and control patient entry into the trial are difficult or impossible to reproduce in clinical practice. This is one of the key reasons for the current emphasis on *outcomes* studies that are conducted in a more typical practice environment. Outcomes studies provide higher levels of external validity because they involve the types of patients and the kind of care that can be provided in routine practice.

For a more detailed question, the pharmacist should include a brief summary of evidence to support the recommendation. The research example at the end of this chapter illustrates a detailed response that might be used in a more formal consultation for a therapeutic recommendation. This example is certainly not typical of most questions that pharmacists currently respond to, but is intended to demonstrate a detailed response. (It should also be noted that it is not reasonable to be expected to provide this level of consultation without a fee.)

COMMUNICATING THE RESPONSE

The response to a drug information question is usually provided verbally, either in person or by telephone, especially if the response is relatively simple. When the response is more complex, as in the research example on page 190, a verbal summary could be appropriate, but the level of detail would require a written response to confirm the verbal information.

When communicating recommendations in response to a drug information question, the information must be provided in the appropriate level of detail and the language used must be appropriate both for the recipient of the information and for its intended purpose. The pharmacist should anticipate and be prepared for additional questions that may arise from the initial response. As stated earlier in this chapter, if the right question is clearly formulated, the need for additional information should be limited.

DOCUMENTATION AND FOLLOW-UP

When documenting pharmaceutical care activities, as described in Chapter 6, pharmacists should also document any drug information provided and recommendations associated with the response. Keeping track of the sources used is helpful in case the pharmacist later needs to do additional investigation.

Whether the pharmacist needs to follow up after supplying a response to a drug information request, and when that follow-up should occur, depends on the situation and is essentially a judgment call. The purpose of follow-up is to find out if the recommendations have been accepted, if there are any further questions, and how the patient has responded to therapy. This information can then be used to determine whether further modifications are needed in the therapeutic plan.

BASIC DRUG INFORMATION LIBRARY

Pharmacists should have access to key references to answer questions within the following categories:
- Adverse drug reactions,
- Compounding/manufacturing,
- Contraindications,
- Disease information,
- Dosage,
- Drug interactions,
- Identification of tablets, foreign drugs, etc.,
- Intravenous compatibility/stability,
- Pharmacokinetics,
- Poison/toxicology,
- Pregnancy/lactation,
- Therapeutic choices.

Many references are useful for multiple categories of information. Electronic drug information databases, and the networks that provide access to these databases, can equip pharmacists with a wide range of drug information resources. For a listing of effective reference works (there are far too many to describe here), refer to *Module 2, Evaluating Drug Literature,* in the Drug Information Series published by the American Society of Health-System Pharmacists (first item in the box on page 184). It contains

LEVELS OF EVIDENCE

The Evidence Based Working Group from McMaster has described a hierarchy of research called the "levels of evidence."[5] They list research designs in order from the most to least valid evidence of treatment efficacy. Following is a modification of that list:

- Level I: Randomized controlled trials or a meta-analysis in which the lower limit of the confidence interval for the treatment effect exceeds the minimal clinically important difference. A meta-analysis—a systematic collection of all available evidence on a question—involves specialized statistical procedures to combine the results of the various studies.

- Level II: Randomized controlled trials or meta-analysis in which the confidence interval for the treatment effect overlaps the minimal clinically important benefit. This type of result indicates possible benefit but does not exclude the possibility that the benefit is clinically insignificant.

- Level III: Nonrandomized concurrent cohort comparisons between patients who did and did not receive therapy. These are the "outcomes" type of studies.

- Level IV: Nonrandomized historical cohort studies in which the comparison is made between current patients who received therapy and patients in the past who did not receive therapy.

- Level V: Nonrandomized historical case control trials. The comparison is made between individuals (the cases) who develop an outcome (such as a disease or disease event like stroke), and patients (the controls) who do not have the outcome. Specified risk factors are identified in the patients' records prior to development of the event. If the presence of risk factors is significantly different between the cases and controls, it indicates an association between the risk factor and the outcome. Case control studies are not used to evaluate treatment efficacy but may identify possible adverse effects of therapy. Case control trials are also useful to study rare outcomes or outcomes that develop only a long time after an exposure.

- Level VI: Case series without controls. A case series may contain useful information about the clinical course and prognosis but cannot provide valid information about efficacy.

- Level VII: Expert opinion. In the absence of specific evidence of efficacy and safety, experts make judgments based on animal data, pharmacology data, or extrapolation of results from similar therapies. This type of evidence is essentially a working hypothesis.

a detailed matrix of secondary and tertiary literature resources. The text *Drug Information: A Guide for Pharmacists* by Malone et al. (second item in the box below) has a section on drug information resources that is a helpful guide for organizing a drug information library.

Recent surveys of community pharmacists indicate that more than 80% of their drug information questions can be answered with previous

USEFUL RESOURCES FOR EVALUATING THE LITERATURE

- Smith GH, Norton LL, Ferrill MJ. *The ASHP Clinical Skills Program Drug Information Module 2: Evaluating Drug Literature.* Bethesda, MD: American Society of Health-System Pharmacists; 1995.

- Mosdell KW. Literature evaluation. In: Malone PM, Mosdell KW, Kier KL, Stanovich JE. *Drug Information: A Guide for Pharmacists.* Stamford, CT: Appleton & Lange; 1996: 89-119.

- Kier KL. Clinical application of statistical analysis. In: Malone PM, Mosdell KW, Kier KL, Stanovich JE. *Drug Information: A Guide for Pharmacists.* Stamford, CT: Appleton & Lange; 1996: 121-49.

- Gehlbach SH. *Interpreting the Medical Literature.* 3rd ed. New York: McGraw-Hill Inc; 1993.

- Riegelman RK, Hirsch RP. *Studying a Study and Testing a Test: How to Read the Science Literature.* 3rd ed. Boston: Little Brown and Company; 1996.

- Hulley SB, Cummings SR, eds. *Designing Clinical Research: An Epidemiological Approach.* Baltimore: Williams & Wilkins; 1988.

- Sackett DL, Richardson WS, Rosenberg W, Haynes RB. *Evidence-Based Medicine: How to Practice and Teach EBM.* New York: Churchill Livingstone; 1997.

- Spilker B. *Guide to Clinical Trials.* New York: Raven Press; 1991.

- The evidence-based medicine web sites: http://cebm.jr2.ox.ac.uk/ and http://hiru.mcmaster.ca/.

- The Cochrane Review Methodology Database in the Cochrane Library, Vista, CA: Update Software Inc; 1997 issue 4.

- Angaran D, panel chair. *Pharmacotherapy Self-Assessment Program Module 5. Biostatistics, Research Design and Literature Evaluation.* Kansas City, MO: American College of Clinical Pharmacy; 1995.

- Drummond R. How to report randomized controlled trials: the CONSORT statement. *JAMA.* 1996;276: 649.

- Begg C, Cho M, Eastwood S, et al. Improving the quality of reporting of randomized controlled trials: the CONSORT statement. *JAMA.* 1996; 276:637-9.

- The Asilomar working group on recommendations for reporting of clinical trials in the biomedical literature. Checklist of information for inclusion in reports of clinical trials. *Ann Intern Med.* 1996;124:741-3.

- Mulrow C, Cook D, series eds. Systematic reviews: synthesis of best evidence for clinical decisions. *Ann Intern Med.* 1997;126:376-80.

knowledge and standard textbooks like *Drug Facts and Comparisons, USP DI,* and *Drug Interaction Facts.* However, as pharmacists continue to build pharmaceutical care practices, the questions will change and the need for access to specialized references and primary literature will increase.

In developing a drug information library, an organized approach maximizes the investment. The pharmacist may wish to contact the closest drug information center affiliated with a college of pharmacy, large hospital, or other institution[6] for advice. It is worthwhile to spend time in a center with drug information experts and ask them to demonstrate and explain the references they use most. Those pharmacists unable to visit a drug information center should visit a college of pharmacy library or a medical library and get advice from the information experts there.

Pharmacists should choose references within their budget and consider if their practice site has any specialized information needs, such as a significant number of cases involving pediatric patients, dermatology, oncology, geriatrics, parenteral drug use, or home care.

Computerization has dramatically increased the ability to sort through vast amounts of medical and pharmaceutical evidence to find specific information for drug therapy decisions. Most practicing pharmacists were not exposed to these types of resources during their formal training. The current climate of heath care consumerism is increasing patient demand for more detailed information about disease states and the risks and benefits of treatment options. Pharmacists and other health care providers will be increasingly challenged to stay current with the evidence for these therapies.

As stated by Edward J. Huth, M.D., former editor of the *Annals of Internal Medicine,* "The strength of a profession lies in its expert generation of information and better management of it than other social groups." Pharmacists' efforts to sharpen their drug information management skills will ensure that they maintain significant roles in the drug therapy decision-making process, and in assisting patients to ensure the best use and outcome from their medications.

REFERENCES

1. American Society of Health-System Pharmacists. ASHP guidelines on the provision of medication information by pharmacists. *Am J Health-Syst Pharm.* 1996;53:1843-5.

2. Troutman WG. Consensus-derived objectives for drug information education. *Drug Inf J.* 1994;28:791-6.

3. Sackett DL, Rosenberg WMC, Gray JAM, et al. Evidence-based medicine: what it is and what it isn't. *BMJ.* 1996;312:71-2.

4. Lowe HJ, Barnett GO. Understanding and using the medical subject headings (MeSH) vocabulary to perform literature searches. *JAMA*. 1994;271:1103-8.

5. Cook DJ, Guyatt GH, Laupacis A, et al. Clinical recommendations using levels of evidence for antithrombotic agents. *Chest*. 1995;108:227S-30S.

6. Rosenberg JM, Fuentes RJ, Starr CH, et al. Pharmacist-operated drug information centers in the United States. *Am J Health-Syst Pharm*. 1995;52:991-6.

BACKGROUND INFORMATION TO OBTAIN FOR PATIENT-SPECIFIC DRUG INFORMATION QUESTIONS

The following is a general guide to additional information the pharmacist may want to request when receiving and defining a specific drug information question. Not all questions would be relevant to all cases, and sometimes further questions may be needed that are not reflected here. Certain facts about the patient, such as age, height, weight, gender, medications, illnesses, known drug allergies, and so on, should be part of the routine patient record that the pharmacist maintains, and are important background for all drug information questions.

ADVERSE DRUG REACTIONS

*   Specific description of the signs and symptoms, severity, and time of onset;

*   Laboratory tests that have been performed to assess the reaction (e.g., serum creatinine, liver function);

*   Any history of a similar reaction to the same medication or one in the same pharmacologic class;

*   Any changes in the medication profile: new drugs, changed dose, discontinued drugs, nonprescription, or herbal products;

*   Current problem list and past medical history;

*   Therapy that has been provided to treat the reaction.

CONTRAINDICATIONS

*   Intended use of medication;

*   Alternative drugs used in past or to consider now;

*   Current and past medical conditions;

*   Current and past medication history;

*   Current and past adverse drug reactions.

DOSAGE

*   Intended use of medication;

*   Any known adverse reactions or sensitivities to medications;

*   Any factors that would affect pharmacokinetics of the drug;

*   Current and past illnesses and medications.

DRUG INTERACTIONS

*   Whether an adverse drug reaction has already occurred;

*   Suspected medications involved;

*   Intended use of medications;

*   Any therapy for the reaction or changes in therapy already initiated;

*   Dosage of medications.

BACKGROUND INFORMATION TO OBTAIN FOR PATIENT-SPECIFIC DRUG INFORMATION QUESTIONS *(CONTINUED)*

THERAPEUTIC CHOICES OR EFFICACY

- Indication for medication;
- Past response to medication for this indication;
- Past response to other medications in general;
- Any known drug allergies or sensitivities.

INTRAVENOUS COMPATIBILITY

- Intended method of administration: piggyback, mix in syringe, large-volume solution, push;
- Concentration, rate of administration, and dosing schedule of other medications;
- Number and type of intravenous lines or sites available;
- Considerations for alternate routes of administration;
- Storage conditions if not to be given immediately.

LACTATION

- Age of infant, weight, general health, current medications, medical conditions;
- Intended use of medication for mother;
- Dosage route, dose, schedule, duration of therapy;
- Other medications and medical conditions of the mother.

PHARMACOKINETICS

- Current renal and hepatic function, any recent changes;
- Any drug levels taken, the timing of the levels, and dosing;

- Other patient-specific details known to alter clearance, volume of distribution, protein binding, sites of distribution, absorption, metabolism;
- Route of administration;
- Any specific reason for questioning kinetics, such as an adverse reaction or lack of therapeutic response.

PREGNANCY

- Whether the patient is already pregnant and if so, what week;
- Whether the medication has already been taken, and how much over what time period;
- Indication for the medication;
- Current and past medical and medication history.

PRODUCT AVAILABILITY OR PRODUCT IDENTIFICATION

- Name and spelling of medication in question;
- Where current information about the medication came from;
- Origination of drug—U.S. or foreign;
- Indication for the medication;
- Physical description of the product if available: shape, size, color markings, code numbers, tablet, capsule, injectable, etc.;
- Whether the product has already been taken and any reactions;
- Where the product was obtained.

SAMPLE DRUG INFORMATION QUESTION RECORD

REQUESTOR: _____

DATE: _____ TIME: _____

WHEN RESPONSE IS NEEDED: _____

REQUESTOR'S STATUS

☐ Physician

☐ Nurse

☐ Hospital or HMO Pharmacist

☐ Community Pharmacist

☐ Consumer

☐ Other: _____

REQUESTOR'S ADDRESS/PHONE:

_____

_____

_____

_____

_____

PATIENT BACKGROUND INFORMATION

Age: _____ Sex: M _____ F _____ Race: _____

Height: _____ Weight: _____

Test Results (Specify type, such as creatinine clearance or liver function):

_____

_____

_____

_____

Chronic Conditions: _____

_____

_____

Acute Conditions: _____

_____

_____

Medications:

Drug	Dose/Frequency	Start Date/Stop Date

QUESTION

_____

_____

_____

_____

SEARCH STRATEGY
Tertiary Resources: _____

_____

_____

_____

Secondary Resources: _____

_____

_____

_____

Other Resources/Contacts: _____

_____

_____

_____

INDEX
Drug Terms: _____

_____

_____

_____

Disease Terms: _____

_____

_____

_____

Descriptors: _____

_____

_____

_____

ANSWER TEXT
Answer Conclusion: _____

_____

_____

_____

References: _____

_____

_____

Response Date: _____ Time Required: _____

Articles Provided: _____

_____

Completed by:_____

RESEARCH EXAMPLE

A patient comes into the pharmacy with a prescription for ranitidine 150 mg, three times a day. He is 42 years old and is being treated for gastroesophageal reflux disease (GERD); he has no other medical problems. During the interview he reports that for the last six months he has been taking ranitidine 150 mg twice daily alternating every other month with omeprazole 20 mg daily. He says that his heartburn symptoms are controlled well during the months that he takes omeprazole, but one to two weeks into the month on ranitidine, his heartburn comes back, and by the end of the month he is miserable. He wants to know if the pharmacist thinks an increase in the ranitidine dose to three times a day will be enough to prevent the problems he has had in the past.

INITIAL PATIENT ADVICE

The pharmacist explains to the patient that the severity of GERD symptoms can vary over time and that an individual patient's response to medications may vary. The pharmacist also says that in some cases increasing the dose of a medication like ranitidine will improve the results. The pharmacist suggests that he try an antacid as needed when he has heartburn and explains the importance of diet, alcohol, smoking, and other lifestyle effects on the severity of GERD. Next, the pharmacist offers to review the literature on treatments for GERD and then provide a recommendation to him and his physician.

Following this discussion with the patient, the pharmacist contacts his physician and learns that the patient has been evaluated by endoscopy and has Grade II esophagitis without stricture, and no evidence of Barrett's esophagus or bleeding. (Note: If specific diagnostic testing had not been done at this point, it would be appropriate to suggest further evaluation prior to continuing empiric therapy.)

THERAPY RECOMMENDATION

The preferred therapy for this patient would be to continue omeprazole 20 mg daily for a total of 12 months. If the patient's symptoms remain well controlled for the remainder of the 12 months, it would then be reasonable to stop therapy. If relapse occurs during therapy or after discontinuation, additional evaluation would be needed to consider possible long-term therapy, higher dose therapy, combination therapy with a promotility drug, or surgery. (Note: Many questions regarding long-term maintenance therapy of GERD are unresolved. Data from additional controlled trials are needed.)

For patients with esophagitis of Grade II or higher, several controlled trials have demonstrated that omeprazole is superior to the histamine-2 receptor antagonists for initial healing and for maintaining remission. The product labeling for omeprazole originally contained a boxed warning regarding the development of gastric carcinoid tumors in rats and recommended that therapy be limited to four to eight weeks. However, the boxed warning has been changed to a precaution, and, based on 12-month trials, the FDA has approved the indication of omeprazole for maintenance therapy. Additional safety data on the long-term use of omeprazole have been published; also, published evaluations of cost-effectiveness in the treatment of Grade II or higher esophagitis have favored omeprazole.

LITERATURE SUPPORT FOR RECOMMENDATION

Practice Guideline: The American College of Gastroenterology (ACG) recently published recommended guidelines for diagnosing and treating GERD.[1] These guidelines represent an extensive review of the literature and consensus recommendations that are very helpful for patient care decision-making. The majority of patients with typical symptoms of uncomplicated GERD may be successfully treated with diet and lifestyle changes, antacids, and/or standard doses of histamine-2 receptor antagonists. For patients with persistent symptoms following empiric therapy, further diagnostic evaluation is recommended. Provided in the ACG guidelines is a summary table of the results of 33 randomized trials of acid suppression therapy for GERD. The results of these trials clearly demonstrate greater efficacy of omeprazole compared to the histamine antagonists for acute healing. In regard to maintenance therapy, the guidelines review several options with clear support for use of chronic proton pump therapy.

Comparative Trials for Maintenance Efficacy: Smith and colleagues[2] conducted a 12-month randomized trial of omeprazole 20 mg daily versus ranitidine 150 mg twice daily in 366 patients with an esophageal stricture due to reflux. Omeprazole was more effective than ranitidine in preventing stricture recurrence, with 30% of omeprazole patients requiring redilatation versus 46% of ranitidine patients ($p<0.01$). Symptom relief was also greater with omeprazole than with ranitidine.

Hallerback and colleagues[3] conducted a 12-month randomized trial of omeprazole 20 mg daily versus 10 mg daily versus ranitidine 150 mg twice daily in 392 patients with healed acute erosive or ulcerative esophagitis (mostly Grade II). The proportion of patients in remission after 12 months was 72% for the 20 mg omeprazole, 62% for the 10 mg omeprazole, and 45% for the ranitidine group. Both the 10 mg and 20 mg doses of omeprazole were significantly better than ranitidine. There was a slight increase in serum gastrin levels in the 20 mg omeprazole group compared to the level after the healing phase (which was achieved with 20 mg to 40 mg omeprazole daily). However, the gastrin levels remained below 100 pmol/L in most patients. Histologic assessment of the gastric mucosa indicated no dysplastic or neoplastic changes.

Dent and colleagues[4] studied omeprazole 20 mg daily versus 20 mg given three consecutive days per week, versus ranitidine 150 mg twice daily for 12 months, for the prevention of relapse in 159 patients after healing with omeprazole. After 12 months the proportion of patients in remission in the omeprazole 20 mg daily group was 89% compared to 32% for "weekend" omeprazole, and 25% for ranitidine. Median gastrin concentrations were increased in the acute healing phase but remained in the normal range and did not change significantly during maintenance treatment. Gastric biopsy taken at healing, and at 6 months and 12 months of maintenance, showed no significant pathologic changes.

Safety of Chronic Omeprazole: Klinkenberg-Knol[5] reported the results of open treatment of 91 patients with daily omeprazole for up to 64 months (mean 48 months) for preventing relapse of reflux esophagitis. Median gastrin levels increased from 60 ng/L to 162 ng/L. Ten of the 91 patients demonstrated very high gastrin levels (>500 ng/L); however, there were influential factors besides therapy with omeprazole. There was an increase of micronodular argyrophil cell hyperplasia and subatrophic or atrophic gastritis, but no dysplasia or neoplasia in any of the biopsy specimens. Follow-up work by this group[6] suggests that atrophic gastritis and argyrophil cell hyperplasia may occur in patients who are positive for helicobacter pylori but not in those who are negative. They suggest that screening for and treating helicobacter pylori prior to long-term use of omeprazole may reduce the risk for atrophy and argyrophil cell hyperplasia.

Skoutakis, in a review of the role of omeprazole in the treatment of GERD,[7] reports that long-term studies have not revealed a trend toward increased incidence of carcinoma of the stomach. They also report that gastric biopsies of more than 5,600 patients receiving long-term omeprazole have shown some hyperplasia of normal gastric cells, but no dysplasia or neoplasia. Astra Merck reports that more than 20 million patients worldwide have been treated with omeprazole.

RESEARCH EXAMPLE REFERENCES

1. DeVault KR, Castell DO. Guidelines for the diagnosis and treatment of gastroesophageal reflux disease. *Arch Intern Med.* 1995;155:2165-73.

2. Smith PM, Kerr GD, Cockel R, et al. A comparison of omeprazole and ranitidine in the prevention of recurrence of benign esophageal stricture. *Gastroenterology.* 1994;107:1312-8.

3. Hallerback B, Unge P, Carling L, et al. Omeprazole or ranitidine in long-term treatment of reflux esophagitis. *Gastroenterology.* 1994;107:1305-11.

4. Dent J, Yeomans ND, Mackinnon M, et al. Omeprazole vs. ranitidine for prevention of relapse in reflux oesophagitis. A controlled double blind trial of their efficacy and safety. *Gut.* 1994;35:590-8.

5. Klinkenberg-Knol EL, Festen HP, Jansen MJ, et al. Long-term treatment with omeprazole for refractory reflux esophagitis: efficacy and safety. *Ann Int Med.* 1994;121:161-7.

6. Kuipers EJ, Lundell L, Klinkenberg-Knol EL, et al. Atrophic gastritis and helicobacter pylori infection in patients with reflux esophagitis treated with omeprazole or fundoplication. *N Engl J Med.* 1996;334:1018-22.

7. Skoutakis VA, Joe RH, Hara DS. Comparative role of omeprazole in the treatment of gastroesophageal reflux disease. *Ann Pharmacother.* 1995;29:1252-62.

Chapter 12

♦

Barriers to Pharmaceutical Care

Change is hard for everyone. Undeniably, pharmacists whose practices are undergoing a transition to pharmaceutical care experience difficulty. A general model for change,[1] which applies to the process pharmacists have experienced in embracing pharmaceutical care, involves these steps:

1. Preparation: Contact ⟹ Awareness.
2. Acceptance: Understanding ⟹ Positive Perception.
3. Commitment: Installation ⟹ Adoption ⟹ Institutionalization ⟹ Internalization.

In this model, there is an initial phase during which pharmacists prepare for the changes ahead, first encountering the term pharmaceutical care and developing an awareness of its existence. During the second phase, pharmacists gradually develop a true understanding of what it means to practice pharmaceutical care and come to view it as a positive force in pharmacy. During the third phase, pharmacists truly begin to change. They make an initial attempt to convert the practice to pharmaceutical care. After this trial period, the new practice is adopted more widely until it becomes part of the usual practice in that pharmacy. Finally, the practice of pharmaceutical care becomes so ingrained and automatic that it has been internalized by the pharmacists and staff and is now part of their newly adopted goals and values.

The initial trial installation of pharmaceutical care usually goes fairly smoothly, but the later phases of change, in which the new practice must become automatic, cause problems for many pharmacists. Even when change is viewed as a positive force, it is difficult to accomplish.

A variety of factors may cause pharmacists to resist changing to pharmaceutical care. They may feel a personal loss from their traditional role and the security that role brought them. They may be concerned about losing traditional standing and position, which is one of the risks of change. Some may see no need to change. They may underestimate the seriousness of problems in the current system; they may be comfortable with their current level of dissatisfaction; or they may view their situation as unchangeable. These pharmacists may view proposed changes as doing more harm than good. Profitability issues and the additional expenses of making the transition to a pharmaceutical care practice may intimidate these pharmacists because they threaten the survival of the pharmacy.

For some pharmacists, resistance may be sparked by the fact that change is being imposed by the marketplace; they feel compelled to implement pharmaceutical care because of decreased profit margins. They feel frustrated that they must react by altering their practice and that they have no real input into changes in the system. Last of all, some pharmacists fear that the costs of change—financial, social, personal, and psychological—may not be outweighed by the perceived benefits.

> **ATTITUDINAL OBSTACLES**
>
> The following problems can interfere with a pharmacist's ability to provide pharmaceutical care:
>
> 1. Inadequate comprehension of what it is and what it entails,
> 2. Misconceptions and false assumptions,
> 3. Fears related to changing roles,
> 4. Lack of personal motivation.

Although several articles have been published about barriers to pharmaceutical care in a variety of settings, little has been written about barriers in the community setting.[2-4] We have grouped the factors listed above and others that impede the pharmacist's ability to implement pharmaceutical care into six categories:

1. Pharmacists' attitudes,
2. Lack of advanced practice skills,
3. Resource-related constraints,
4. System-related constraints,
5. Intraprofessional obstacles,
6. Academic/educational obstacles.

PHARMACISTS' ATTITUDES

Attitude is a critical barrier to overcome. Unfortunately, some pharmacists are reluctant to accept the inevitable changes in the profession. Some lack confidence in their abilities to implement a pharmaceutical care practice. Others are uncommitted to making the necessary changes. Some pharmacists are pessimistic about whether pharmacy can remain a viable profession in general, and some fear that delegating dispensing tasks to technicians will make pharmacists obsolete. Discussed below are four general attitudinal obstacles a pharmacist must address to ensure the success of a pharmaceutical care practice.

LACK OF COMPREHENSION

Although pharmaceutical care has been discussed extensively in the field since 1987, many pharmacists do not understand the full concept. A working definition of pharmaceutical care should include the activities discussed earlier in this book:

- Establishing a therapeutic relationship with the patient,
- Interviewing the patient to collect data needed to identify drug therapy problems,
- Developing and implementing a patient-specific care plan to resolve identified problems,
- Providing ongoing monitoring and follow-up services to the patient,
- Documenting all patient care activities.

When pharmacists understand the definition of pharmaceutical care, they grasp more thoroughly the reality of changing their practice focus from dispensing a tangible drug product to providing both tangible and intangible services associated with patient care.

MISCONCEPTIONS

Common beliefs about pharmaceutical care that can prevent pharmacists from creating a successful practice include:

1. Pharmacists have already been practicing pharmaceutical care for their entire careers.
2. Patients will not accept this type of care or be willing to pay for it.
3. Pharmaceutical care will create "turf wars" with other health care providers.

The first belief is false for the vast majority of pharmacists. Pharmaceutical care includes follow-up and documentation of activities with patients, which is rarely done in a traditional practice. Additionally, many community pharmacists do not create patient charts that contain important patient history information for identifying and treating problems. Pharmaceutical care requires more patient counseling and data collection than pharmacists typically do, and also requires pharmacists to accept responsibility for their patients' drug therapy. Simply acting as an advisor in a casual sense is not pharmaceutical care.

The second item in the list is a very common misconception. True, some patients will feel that they do not require pharmaceutical care, and some will not consider it a service worth paying for, but this can be said of all goods and services sold anywhere. Nationally, there are successful pharmaceutical care practices that charge and receive payment for pharmaceutical care services. The perceived value of these services will grow over time, as patients realize the benefits of pharmaceutical care and tell others. In the meantime, pharmacists should target markets of consumers who accept the value of this care and are willing to pay for it. By identifying the needs of the consumers, a pharmacist can respond by offering a service that satisfies the need.

Regarding the third belief, pharmaceutical care can actually be used as a bridge to develop professional relationships with physicians and other health care providers. In fact, when pharmacists concentrate on establishing professional relationships with other health care providers, the potential for "turf wars" subsides. Hostility occurs only when a physician or prescriber infers that the pharmacist is criticizing the prescriber's decisions or prescribing habits.

To avoid misconceptions among other health care providers, pharmacists must let them know that:

- Pharmacists have information that physicians can use.
- Pharmacists are interested in working cooperatively with the physician to achieve the physician's outcomes and goals for the patient.
- Pharmacists see patients more often than physicians, and therefore can act as screeners for patient problems. As problems are identified, the physician will be informed and included in all decisions.
- Due to their accessibility in the community, pharmacists can provide patient education services deemed necessary by the physician.

Problems between pharmacists and physicians often develop because the pharmacist has tried to explain the process to the physician without fully understanding it first. If this is the case, it may be necessary for the pharmacist to re-explain the concept to the physician and emphasize the benefits to patients, since that is where both parties' true interests lie. The benefits of pharmaceutical care need to be concrete and readily understood by patients and other health care providers.

FEAR OF CHANGE

Some pharmacists allow their fear of changing roles to become an obstacle to practicing pharmaceutical care. Pharmacists may worry that they lack the skills or knowledge to incorporate the concept of pharmaceutical care into their practices. Taking on responsibility for outcomes of a patient's drug therapy can be intimidating and frightening. Because some practitioners never intended to provide this level of care when they entered the field of pharmacy, they feel threatened and reluctant to embrace it.

Fear can be a powerful force in blocking change. If a pharmacist does not see the value in altering his practice, or flatly does not want to change the practice, it is highly unlikely that a change will occur. Pharmaceutical care is not a particularly easy concept to put into effect; doing so means going through a transition period that can be very difficult. Too often, pharmacists in mid-transition revert back to "old" practice strategies instead of fully implementing pharmaceutical care. This wastes time and resources. Inevitably, these practitioners cling to the hope that market conditions will not change dramatically and that the meager profit margins of dispensing will be enough to allow them to stay in business.

To overcome the obstacle of fear, pharmacists must adopt a "one patient at a time" philosophy. The skills and knowledge needed to provide pharmaceutical care will not be gained quickly, but will develop over time. The key to overcoming fears is for pharmacists to believe in their knowledge and abilities. Patient by patient, as pharmacists build a pharmaceutical care practice, they will eventually gain confidence and come to accept change.

LACK OF MOTIVATION

Because of its indeterminate nature, motivation to make a change must arise from within an individual. Perhaps an underlying personality characteristic improves the chances of a person initiating change. Because different people require different motivating factors, such as job satisfaction, professional success, or money, it is difficult to describe one thing that will impel every pharmacist to change to pharmaceutical care. Each one must identify the goals or positive outcomes that will ignite his or her motivation. The success of pharmaceutical care implementation begins and ends with each individual pharmacist.

LACK OF ADVANCED PRACTICE SKILLS

Another important obstacle is a lack of advanced practice skills in therapeutics, clinical problem solving, communication, documentation, and research. Pharmacists need to recognize and feel confident about the skills they already possess and put time and effort into building those that are weak.

THERAPEUTICS

For several reasons, knowledge of therapeutics is inconsistent among practitioners. Surprisingly, number of years in the field or number of years spent studying pharmacy do not appear to be accurate indicators of therapeutic knowledge. Some pharmacists make a career-long commitment to increasing their therapeutic base, while others concentrate on other areas. Those who commit to developing an excellent therapeutics knowledge base typically can identify more problems, identify problems faster, and develop a wider range of potential solutions and care plans. For most pharmacists, the common fear that their knowledge is inadequate to provide pharmaceutical care is usually groundless. Often, they need only to be instructed in how to use and communicate the knowledge they have already gained. Many existing drug therapy problems do not require sophisticated therapeutic solutions. As pharmacists' drug assessment skills improve, they need to expand their therapeutic knowledge, which may be accomplished through programs offered by colleges of pharmacy, accredited continuing education providers, and state and national organizations.

CLINICAL PROBLEM SOLVING

Some pharmacists interested in providing pharmaceutical care feel overwhelmed by their lack of clinical problem-solving skills in therapeutics and pathophysiology. Pharmacists who view their therapeutics as weak should proceed cautiously, but proceed, nevertheless, and gradually build their clinical problem-solving skills, which are essential for providing pharmaceutical care. Clinical problem solving is learnable, but only by practice. Pharmacists who do not develop this skill will fall short when it comes to caring for patients and contributing to the health care team.

Almost every practitioner currently possesses basic problem-solving skills, but not all pharmacists have consistently applied these skills in resolving clinical problems. Once they develop an increased understanding of therapeutics and drug information skills, clinical problem solving becomes less difficult and, with appropriate training and practice, eventually becomes a natural thought process.

An important step is mastering the strategy of asking good questions so it becomes a natural, automatic behavior rather than rehearsed and stilted. Because taking time to practice can become frustrating, some pharmacists become discouraged and stop. It's important to be aware that learning clinical problem-solving skills is time consuming and that patience is essential. Enrolling in courses that teach these skills may be helpful.

COMMUNICATION SKILLS

The most important skill to master in the area of pharmaceutical care is communication. Pharmacists providing care will interact with patients and staff more frequently, in verbal and written communications, than they do in traditional dispensing practices. Collecting patient histories requires interviewing skills that many pharmacists never developed because they did not need to. Strong communication skills are important not only for eliciting key information from patients, but also for marketing and explaining the benefits of pharmaceutical care to patients, third party payers, and other health care providers. These skills are also critical for communicating effectively with physicians and other health care providers about a patient's drug therapy.

As pharmacists implement pharmaceutical care in their practices, there will be an unlimited number of encounters with patients and health care providers. Having good "people skills" will make it easier to incorporate this practice philosophy. On the other hand, those who lack people skills will have a difficult time changing roles. Participating in educational programs and workshops on interpersonal communication is a good way to start improving. Practicing and developing these skills over time is important too. Building communication skills requires a commitment to change and a desire to become a more competent provider.

DOCUMENTATION

Most pharmacists are not accustomed to documenting patient care activities, whereas other health care providers spend a great deal of time on documentation. By documenting their care, they create a tool—patient charts—that can be used to help provide optimal care for their patients. At the same time, they create a record by which they are able to bill for services rendered to patients and third party payers. Limited experience with documentation requirements and systems is a barrier that pharmacists must overcome. Without consistent and efficient documentation, it is difficult to provide optimal care to patients and prove the value of pharmaceutical care to the health care system.

Documentation systems allow pharmacists to systematically review their patients' health status and drug therapy. They also provide an ongoing record of care, including pharmacists' interventions, successes and failures of treatment regimens, care plans implemented, and patient follow-ups. Currently, there are no standard documentation and billing methods available to pharmacists, which may prove to be an obstacle to reimbursement. Because third party payers are likely to want one system in place to ensure consistency among pharmacies, standards will need to be implemented in the future.

Some pharmacists have invested in computer documentation systems to help them keep patient care records. Although these systems are improving, they remain imperfect. As discussed in Chapter 6, pharmacists may be better off initially with a paper system until their patient volume grows and they have time to critically evaluate available computer systems.

DRUG INFORMATION

It is difficult to implement pharmaceutical care without an understanding and knowledge of drug information resources. The drug information library that many pharmacists keep at their practice site is limited. In addition, many pharmacists feel inadequate when it comes to interpreting the literature. Without access to needed references and without the skills to critically evaluate the literature, pharmacists cannot effectively use drug information resources to help them identify and resolve drug therapy problems. Pharmacists can develop drug information skills and confidence in their abilities by enrolling in educational programs through pharmacy schools or self-study courses. They can also subscribe to services that allow electronic access to commonly used drug information databases and can make arrangements with a local or national drug information center to get help with answering difficult drug information questions.

RESOURCE-RELATED CONSTRAINTS

TIME

Some pharmacists are very concerned about the lack of time they have for pharmaceutical care. They may be using a workflow pattern that does not support patient care services or they may be uncomfortable delegating tasks to others. The cost in time and money of additional training may compound these obstacles. It's important to realize that, when implemented, pharmaceutical care will actually save time and enhance the profitability of the pharmacy.

In reality, pharmacists lack time because they concentrate on the wrong activity: dispensing. Could someone else do various tasks more efficiently, quickly, or cheaply? If so, these activities should be delegated. Pharmacists need to be cognizant of how time is spent each day and must prepare a plan for implementing pharmaceutical care, or else they are setting themselves up for unnecessary frustrations and possible failure. A certain amount of time should be routinely scheduled for patient care activities, even if it is just a fraction of each day. Restructuring priorities can allow for extra time, especially in the beginning stages of launching a pharmaceutical care practice. Practitioners should start slowly, with two or three patients per week, then slowly increase the number to an attainable, manageable level. Pharmacists who commit to making the time will find the time for pharmaceutical care.

FINANCES

Financial concerns may be fueled by the false belief that large sums of money are necessary to implement pharmaceutical care. Redesigning the pharmacy, hiring more personnel, and purchasing an expensive computer or documentation system may seem like necessities from the very beginning, but in reality the changes made need not be expensive. Pharmaceutical care is a *practice philosophy* that focuses on the patient—it is not the physical environment or the computer software system. By focusing on the interaction with patients, pharmacists can carefully plan for making changes at a minimal cost as they become necessary. Employing good money management habits will make it easier to add personnel, fixtures, or a documentation system when they are needed.

SPACE

A space dedicated to providing patient care in privacy is critical. Without it, patients may be concerned about confidentiality and may not be willing to provide pharmacists with needed health care information. As mentioned previously, a patient care area does not require expensive pharmacy redesigns. A semiprivate area can be created with just two office partitions placed strategically.

PERSONNEL

To provide pharmaceutical care to patients, pharmacists need to free their time from other functions—which can only be done with the proper use of technicians and auxiliary personnel. Not only is it important to have the right people in place, but each person, including the pharmacist, needs to have a job description that includes their primary and secondary responsibilities. Some jobs and responsibilities may need to be redefined.

All pharmacy personnel must be included in the implementation process. Everyone needs to feel like an important member of the pharmacy team. Input should be welcome from all employees; otherwise, dissension and dissatisfaction may block the progress of the implementation.

MANAGEMENT

Some pharmacists who are truly committed to pharmaceutical care may have their excitement extinguished by lack of management support. Support from managers is essential to hire or retrain personnel, create patient care areas, and update drug information resources. Managers' emotional backing goes a long way to help pharmacists cope with the many changes required to implement pharmaceutical care. Wichman, et al. note that management must consider four key areas[5]:

- Structure and function of the organization,
- Human resources,
- Educational needs,
- Revisions to the system and processes.

The challenge for management is to retain their current profitability while undergoing the changes needed for pharmaceutical care. In some situations, focusing on short-term profitability goals has hindered pharmaceutical care implementation. By not planning for the future and setting long-term goals, the profession faces a real danger of shrinking profits and reduced viability in the marketplace.

SYSTEMS-RELATED CONSTRAINTS

REIMBURSEMENT

Reimbursement issues continue to haunt pharmacy. Of all the obstacles to pharmaceutical care, these seem to be the most real and difficult to overcome. Without some type of payment, it will be financially unfeasible for most, if not all, pharmacists to provide this care over the long term. There are many up-front expenses required to implement pharmaceutical care and, at this time, no consistent or guaranteed way to recoup them. Reimbursement is still based on the drug product. Pharmacy benefit plans offered by third party payers continue to reduce payments for drug products without reimbursing pharmacists for care provided. This offers little incentive for pharmacists to change their practices.

However, the financial value of pharmaceutical care has been suggested by Johnson and Bootman's study of drug mortality and morbidity problems in today's society.[6] Drug-related problems, a real danger to patients, are addressed by pharmaceutical care. Pharmacists should consistently bill patients and third party payers for cognitive services as a way of overcoming reimbursement barriers. Some pharmacists are reluctant to ask patients for direct payment; yet if they do not, patients will not demand coverage of pharmaceutical care services from third party payers and insurers' attitudes will not change. Only when pharmacists start billing consistently for services rendered and documenting the care they have provided will the health care system start recognizing the contributions of pharmacists. Like other health care professions, pharmacy needs to develop universal systems for billing that streamline the process and are recognized and accepted by third party payers.

PATIENT DEMAND

Patients may resist the adoption of pharmaceutical care for many reasons. Some may be reluctant to spend additional time with the pharmacist because they are unfamiliar with the pharmacist's expertise. Some may be concerned about issues related to cost and value. Some patients may even resist pharmaceutical care because they believe the pharmacist is encroaching on their physician's "territory," and they don't want to anger their physician.

Pharmacists definitely should respect the physicians' territory, but at the same time they must assert their claim to a new health care role. By identifying patient needs and explaining to patients how they will benefit from a service, pharmacists can win over reluctant patients. Stressing the cooperative aspects of the pharmacist-patient (therapeutic) relationship will help dispose patients toward accepting pharmaceutical care as part of their health care.

A key reason why patients do not demand pharmaceutical care is that they do not understand the concept. To compound the problem, many pharmacists have little or no experience with marketing and creating marketing plans, which, if done right, can create a demand. Taking business or marketing courses, or hiring marketing firms, can be helpful for developing marketing strategies.

Because individual and local efforts can only do so much, the profession needs to launch a major public relations and education campaign to alter the expectations of patients and create a demand. Ultimately, however, it is only the effective provision of pharmaceutical care that will convince patients and others of its value.

ACCEPTANCE BY NURSES AND PHYSICIANS

Realistically, not all physicians or health care providers will appreciate pharmacists taking on the role of a patient care provider. Nurses, for example, may view drug therapy outcomes as their domain and resist pharmacy's advances in pharmaceutical care. This is a temporary obstacle, however, that can be overcome as pharmacists demonstrate their skill at making rational drug therapy decisions and their ability to collaborate with others on the health care team. Pharmacists should not get discouraged by those health care professionals who see no value in pharmaceutical care. With time, pharmacists will gain trust and respect from most health care providers for their clinical input and their role in health care delivery. To demonstrate their willingness to take on responsibility for their patients' drug therapy, pharmacists must develop close working relationships with other health care providers and provide well-thought-out recommendations to physicians.

LACK OF DATA

The lack of data proving pharmaceutical care's value to society is a major obstacle to its acceptance. Practitioners, national and state associations, and colleges of pharmacy need to coordinate their activities and support outcomes research that provides evidence of pharmaceutical care's merit. Without such research, pharmaceutical care is a hard sell to third party administrators and consumers.

INTRAPROFESSIONAL OBSTACLES

PROFESSIONAL RELATIONSHIPS

In the past, pharmacy organizations representing pharmacists in certain practice settings have not worked together efficiently for the common good of pharmacy. This has fragmented the profession and made it a less unified force in the political arena. If agendas continue to compete, the unity needed for pharmaceutical care to be accepted will be prohibited. Differing terminology and definitions used to describe pharmaceutical care are examples of this fragmentation. In addition, some practitioners and organizations subscribe to the disease management approach to pharmaceutical care, while others embrace a generalist approach. Pharmacists from all practice settings and all pharmacy organizations must cooperate closely to make pharmaceutical care a reality.

BOARDS OF PHARMACY

Pharmacy, like other health care professions, is a dynamic field. As pharmacists' responsibilities change, so does pharmacy practice as a whole. Occasionally, pharmacy board regulations and rules—such as pharmacist-technician ratios and limits on technician activities—impede pharmacists' implementation of pharmaceutical care. Although these impediments are not intentional, they occur because outdated rules remain despite changes in the profession. It is important that state boards, state associations, colleges of pharmacy, and practitioners communicate effectively to address such problems.

COLLEGES OF PHARMACY

Although some colleges of pharmacy may not view themselves as having a role in creating the capacity for pharmaceutical care, their support is essential. Colleges must re-examine their missions and alumni must lobby their colleges for assistance. Pharmacy colleges can give practitioners access to important resources—including educational programs and faculty expertise. They can also carry out key research efforts in areas related to pharmaceutical care and offer students unique opportunities to broaden their skills and perspective.

ACADEMIC AND EDUCATIONAL OBSTACLES

Lack of mentors and role models and the need for curriculum changes are the top obstacles in this category. Pharmacists, like students, learn by watching and emulating the behaviors of role models. In implementing pharmaceutical care, most pharmacists have to figure things out for themselves, since they do not have other experts to follow. Fortunately, this is a temporary obstacle. As more practitioners convert their practices, the number of mentors and role models will increase.

Many pharmacy students who have become aware of pharmaceutical care express disappointment about the lack of mentors providing this care to patients. Colleges of pharmacy can help rectify this problem by supporting innovative practitioners and encouraging them to develop mentoring relationships with students.

Pharmacy students graduating from colleges of pharmacy should know what pharmaceutical care is and how to provide it. Unfortunately, many are intimidated by this level of practice. To compound the problem, some pharmacists are relying on new graduates to lead them into pharmaceutical care rather than taking the lead themselves.

Curricula must be examined closely, and all faculty must gain an understanding of pharmaceutical care as it exists today, as well as how it will evolve in the future. Armed with this understanding, faculty can better show students how pharmaceutical care fits into the practice of pharmacy as a whole. Moving to a student-centered curriculum and emphasizing small-group discussions, problem-solving activities, patient cases, and problem-based learning techniques will help students grasp pharmaceutical care concepts.

Because curricular changes must not be done in a vacuum, practitioners must provide direction and input to colleges. In addition, students must interact with patients and other health care providers earlier in their training to increase their understanding of the health care system and improve their interpersonal, communication, and empathy skills.

With the proper support, good planning, time, and commitment, pharmacists can overcome any obstacles detailed in this chapter. The profession is changing rapidly—out of necessity—and with this change comes opportunity. Pharmacists can have a positive effect on the future of the profession if, instead of fearing change, they embrace it.

REFERENCES

1.   Kirkpatrick DL. *How to Manage Change Effectively.* San Francisco: Jossey-Bass Publishers; 1986:34.

2.   May JR. Barriers to pharmaceutical care in the acute care setting. *Am J Hosp Pharm.* 1993;50:1608-11.

3.   Swift BG. Barriers to pharmaceutical care in the home care setting. *Am J Hosp Pharm.* 1993;50:1611-4.

4.   Louie N, Robertson N. Barriers to pharmaceutical care in the managed care setting. *Am J Hosp Pharm.* 1993;50:1614-7.

5.   Wichman K, Hales B, O'Brodovich M, et al. Management considerations to implementing pharmaceutical care. *Can J Hosp Pharm.* 1993;46:265-7.

6.   Johnson JA, Bootman JL. Drug-related morbidity and mortality and the economic impact of pharmaceutical care. *Am J Health-Syst Pharm.* 1997; 54:554-8.

Chapter 13

◆

Creating the Infrastructure

Many factors, both within and outside the pharmacy, influence the environment and infrastructure necessary to support a successful pharmaceutical care practice. This chapter will explore these factors and their impact.

INTERNAL FACTORS

ATTITUDE OF PHARMACY STAFF

The attitude of the pharmacy staff toward pharmaceutical care is extremely important to the success of a pharmaceutical care practice. A positive outlook and enthusiasm for providing care to patients will help the staff overcome the many obstacles that arise. Before beginning to implement pharmaceutical care, it is important to call a meeting of all staff, including pharmacists, pharmacy technicians, and other support personnel, to explain the importance of offering pharmaceutical care services and the changes that the pharmacy will be undertaking. For staff to support the concept of pharmaceutical care, they must understand its value in helping patients and recognize its importance to the pharmacy's long-term financial survival.

INCENTIVES

During the implementation process, a plan to motivate and reward staff for their pharmaceutical care activities will help drive their progress towards adopting the new practice. In a traditional retail pharmacy, employee pharmacists may receive rewards, such as bonuses, based on profit margins that result from the sale of prescriptions. In the future, the successful pharmaceutical care practice will need an established method to track the staff's performance in providing pharmaceutical care services in order to reward and provide incentives for the staff. Such incentives should be based on the care provided, and not solely on the pharmacy's overall financial performance. Possible incentives include the number of pharmaceutical care services documented, the number of pharmaceutical care claims submitted for billing, or patients' satisfaction with the service. Although pharmacists gain personal satisfaction from helping patients when they provide pharmaceutical care, their efforts should be reinforced by a system of recognition and rewards.

DESIGN AND WORKFLOW

The pharmacy design and workflow must facilitate consistent, efficient, and focused delivery of pharmaceutical care to patients. A private area for patient interviews and counseling, a work area for pharmacists to review patient cases and make phone calls, and space for a pharmaceutical care documentation system must all be identified. A documentation system, either paper or computer, must be established to maintain patient records and keep track of the pharmaceutical care services delivered. The new pharmacy workflow must allow for delivery of pharmaceutical care to patients who choose to receive it as well as for basic dispensing of prescription medications to patients who do not want these additional services.

SUPPORT FROM OTHER STAFF

In many practice settings, support for the pharmaceutical care environment may need to extend to the rest of the business operation. When the pharmacy is located in a large grocery store, for example, it is important to consider how factors in the store's total business operation will affect the pharmaceutical care practice, such as the attitude of managers outside the pharmacy department. All staff, including clerks and shelf stockers, should be able to describe the pharmaceutical care services and direct patients to the pharmacy. Giving an educational presentation during a staff meeting is an effective way to give employees a clear understanding of the pharmaceutical care service.

Ways to give incentives to nonpharmacy managers for their support of pharmaceutical care activities should also be explored. If this is not feasible, at least these managers should not be financially penalized when costs are incurred for implementing pharmaceutical care in their stores.

Keep in mind that the store manager for a large retail business may not understand or appreciate the pharmacy department's professional interest in wanting to offer pharmaceutical care services. Also, the business manager may not want to provide the necessary financial resources for remodeling or adding staff to the pharmacy if these expenses are not offset with revenue generated from the new pharmaceutical care services. This is a difficult issue because the business will likely be required to carry the expenses of implementation for some time before a reasonable revenue stream is created from this newly offered service. Any business that chooses to offer pharmaceutical care must be financially stable to withstand the delay of return on investment.

To obtain the business manager's support, meetings should be held with the pharmacy staff in which the pharmaceutical care services are fully described. These meetings must emphasize short-term and long-term financial potential, as well as the positive impact of pharmaceutical care on customer satisfaction to generate return business.

BUSINESS FLOOR PLAN

The floor plan of the entire retail business operation, how the pharmacy is integrated into it, and competition for space are important considerations. Management must balance the space needs of the pharmaceutical care practice with requirements for merchandising space. The patient care area should be thought through carefully, including how it fits with the workflow of the pharmacy and the rest of the business layout. One way to create the space needed for pharmaceutical care is to identify and discontinue merchandise that sells poorly.

CLIMATE

When pharmaceutical care is implemented, the climate of the pharmacy changes. Patients will begin to perceive the pharmacy as a health care center in which their overall health care needs are addressed, rather than as a retail business at which they simply purchase medications and other health care products. Expectations for patient care service and adjustments in attitude about the time needed to process a prescription will change, as well. A strong marketing effort (see Chapter 9) can facilitate this change in expectations and perceptions of the pharmacy.

EXTERNAL FACTORS

Among the factors that can have a major effect on the success of a pharmaceutical care practice is whether other pharmacies in the community are implementing similar services. If they are, the pharmacist can network with local colleagues about common issues and concerns. In addition, the concept of pharmaceutical care is easier to market to the local public and area health care professionals when it seems to be a common practice in the community's pharmacies.

REGULATIONS

State and federal regulations can play a role in pharmaceutical care by either impairing, prohibiting, or supporting its practice. It is important for state pharmacy boards to recognize pharmaceutical care practice when creating and modifying rules and regulations for the practice of pharmacy. When rules that address traditional pharmacy practice are written, they must be carefully crafted so their adoption will not hamper or prevent the operation of a pharmaceutical care practice. The state board should also be open to allowing special exemptions for new innovative pharmacy practice models that do not conform with existing regulations for traditional practice. For example, the board may need to grant a special licensure exemption for pharmacists who want to deliver a pharmaceutical care service in a physician's office rather than in a traditional pharmacy.

Board of pharmacy rules regarding use of pharmacy technicians should allow prescription preparation duties to be delegated as appropriate so that pharmacists can focus on pharmaceutical care. Legislation or regulation should also be adopted for collaborative practice agreements, allowing pharmacists and physicians to work together using drug therapy management protocols to manage patients' drug-related needs. Additional supportive rules could allow pharmacists to administer medications (e.g., immunizations) and order lab tests when necessary (e.g., drug levels). At the enforcement level, boards of pharmacy could get involved in disciplinary actions with pharmacies that advertise pharmaceutical care services but provide only traditional pharmacy service.

PROFESSIONAL GROUPS

Professional pharmacy organizations can foster a positive pharmaceutical care practice environment by mobilizing the political efforts, financial and educational resources, and administrative expertise necessary to help transform the profession. Professional organizations can have a strong political influence by promoting legislation and regulations that support pharmaceutical care practice.

Professional groups can spearhead public education campaigns to help educate consumers, health care professionals, legislators, and others about the value of pharmaceutical care and the contemporary role of the pharmacist. Because pharmaceutical care involves a team approach to health care delivery, other health care professionals must be made aware of its benefits. Ultimately the goal is not only to gain their support for the concept, but to establish sources of patient referrals for specific services. These public education campaigns can supplement individual pharmacies' local marketing strategies, as well, and can help educate such groups as insurance companies, payers, employers, and employee benefit managers.

Professional organizations can also provide training and educational programs for pharmacists on how to implement pharmaceutical care. Such programs can be coordinated cooperatively with local colleges of pharmacy and, when feasible, could be considered for credit towards a nontraditional Pharm.D. When working with colleges to offer these programs, the associations can provide administrative and promotional support while the college faculty develops the content and provides the instruction. In a collaborative educational initiative, the state association leadership, college deans, and individual faculty members must be committed to pharmaceutical care practice and share a common vision for the future of pharmacy. Collaborative training efforts should be undertaken with an eye toward building the capacity for pharmaceutical care in the local health care system.

Examples of state-level efforts are the Iowa Center for Pharmaceutical Care (a partnership of the Iowa Pharmacists Association, the Iowa Pharmacy Foundation, the University of Iowa College of Pharmacy, and Drake University College of Pharmacy and Health Sciences) and the California Center for Pharmaceutical Care (a partnership of the California Pharmacists Association and the pharmacy colleges at the University of Southern California and the University of the Pacific).

> ### KEY ELEMENTS FOR SUCCESSFUL PHARMACEUTICAL CARE IMPLEMENTATION
>
> - Positive attitude of pharmacy staff and other employees and managers in the facility;
> - Incentives to motivate and reward staff;
> - Proper pharmacy design, workflow, and allocation of space in the facility;
> - Promotion of a professional health care climate in the pharmacy;
> - State and federal regulations that support rather than impede pharmaceutical care efforts;
> - Political, educational, and administrative support from professional pharmacy organizations;
> - Collaborative training arrangements with colleges of pharmacy;
> - Formation of networks to offer pharmaceutical care services and enter into contracts with employers and payers;
> - Strong leadership from innovative practitioners.

State pharmacy associations can work with the colleges to prepare pharmacy students for pharmaceutical care practice and help develop practice sites where students can get basic, hands-on experience in pharmaceutical care. As students become comfortable and skilled in delivering pharmaceutical care, they can create more in-depth services and tools for the pharmacy to use. For example, students with advanced skills have developed protocols for a specific service, such as immunizations, and have designed interactive patient education tools for such diseases as hypertension. From their exposure to advanced-level students and the college faculty who supervise them, pharmacists at these sites enhance their own expertise, as well. In essence, the interface between practice and education benefits both groups and helps further the development of the pharmaceutical care practice.

Professional associations can also work collaboratively with college faculty to initiate practice-based research projects to demonstrate the value of pharmacists' contributions to health care, to learn more about the process of implementing pharmaceutical care, or to gather pharmacoeconomic and outcomes-related data. Results of projects and studies can be applied locally and across the country to help demonstrate the value of pharmaceutical care and to support efforts to receive payment for these services.

NETWORKS

Forming networks of pharmacies that offer pharmaceutical care services is a way to generate enthusiasm among a broad base of practitioners and to speed the progress of implementation. When networks exist, they can enter into pharmaceutical care benefit contracts with insurers, payers, or employers. It's important for employers and benefit managers to understand the value of pharmaceutical care so that they demand it for their employees. Likewise, payers must recognize its impact on total medical cost savings as well as its positive effect on the quality of life and productivity of clients and employees. Even without a network or contract, insurers and payers can affect the pharmaceutical care environment by their willingness, or unwillingness, to pay for individual claims submitted for pharmaceutical care services.

CONCLUSION

As a whole, the factors reviewed in this chapter will have a synergistic effect in establishing the right environment for pharmaceutical care. The most important element, however, is the leadership of several innovative practitioners who are willing to take risks and initiate the transition from product-focused to patient-focused practice. As they experience positive results, other pharmacists will be encouraged to follow. Much will be learned from the hard work of these dedicated pioneers. Momentum will build until, eventually, pharmaceutical care is implemented across the entire profession.

Chapter 14

◆

Developing a Practice Implementation Plan

A comprehensive implementation plan is essential when making the transition from a dispensing-oriented practice to a pharmaceutical care practice. Without an action plan, the number of issues can seem overwhelming and the effort is likely to be disorganized. To improve the chances for a successful transition, pharmacists should invest sufficient time and resources at the outset so they can proceed in a coordinated fashion and evaluate their progress along the way.

In Stephen Covey's best-selling book, *The Seven Habits of Highly Effective People*, one of his recommendations is to "begin with the end in mind."[1] Not surprisingly, this principle rings true in nearly any situation in which change is sought. In the case of pharmaceutical care, clearly defining the desired patient services and envisioning the specifics of the future practice will help confirm when the new practice and related services are actually in place.

But what exactly is a pharmaceutical care practice? How will such a practice be carried out? What patients will receive care? How much will be charged to provide the service? What resources and organizational infrastructure will be needed to support the service? All these questions and more must be answered before a plan can be put in action.

EVALUATE GOALS

Although implementing a pharmaceutical care practice can be extremely challenging, it has the potential to be a very rewarding experience. Pharmacists who decide to embark on such a journey should carefully evaluate both their professional and their financial goals. Because investments in time, energy, and money will be required, setting attainable and measurable goals related to pharmaceutical care should be top priority. Is the objective to enhance professional fulfillment, increase pharmacy revenue, elevate the health care image of the pharmacy, or perhaps even facilitate pharmacist recruitment efforts? Whatever the nature of the general goal, it should be stated in terms that can be measured. Examples of goals that are stated appropriately appear in the box below. If the goal is simply to provide pharmaceutical care to patients, it should include, at minimum, a measurable reference to the number of patients who will receive the service and the projected revenue from the service over a defined period of time.

EXAMPLES OF CLEARLY DEFINED GOALS

1. Increase nonprescription professional revenue for the pharmacy by 50% over the next 12 months.

2. Increase the number of patients seeking pharmacist advice by 25%.

3. Reduce the length of time to recruit new pharmacy staff by 50%.

IDENTIFY SERVICES

Once the overall goals have been established, the next step is to determine exactly what types of services the patients and other marketplace stakeholders will find most valuable. First, assess the current patient population served by the pharmacy. Are patients primarily older and retired, with chronic medical conditions? Or are they young married couples with children in generally good health? The types of services for each group are naturally quite different.

Second, identify the types of medical conditions and drug therapies most commonly seen in patients who frequent the pharmacy or among the major age groups in the pharmacy's service area. Also, pinpoint the prescribers who represent the bulk of prescriptions processed by the pharmacy and the medical specialties they practice. By researching the overall demographics and disease prevalence within the pharmacy's service area, it is possible to begin assessing the market growth potential for a given type of service. If the current and potential patient populations are not assessed, there is a big risk of developing services related to a specific professional interest of the pharmacist, only to discover that demand is minimal and potential for new business development is limited.

A TEAM EFFORT

When the decision to implement pharmaceutical care comes from the pharmacy owner or manager—as is most often the case—it is critical to solicit input and cooperation from the entire pharmacy staff. If a staff-level pharmacist wishes to implement the new service, obtaining management support and the cooperation of other staff is equally important. In any case, the greater the team effort, the greater the success potential.

Before proceeding beyond the goal-setting and service-definition stages, all members of the pharmacy team should be assembled to discuss the goals of the new service and how each individual can contribute to reaching those goals. This is really a marketing activity: inevitably, certain members will not understand the need or desire for change and will need to be sold on the idea. The person leading the implementation effort must be prepared to overcome objection and inspire the group to undertake the challenges ahead.

During the initial meeting, the steps involved in implementing pharmaceutical care should be outlined. This is also an appropriate time to ask individuals with key skills to assume responsibility for specific activities. Involving everyone from the beginning will enhance adoption of the new practice and infuse the implementation plan with a greater number of ideas and perspectives.

ACTION PLAN

The activities described in this section should be included in the implementation action plan and discussed at the initial staff meeting of the pharmacy. A suggested timetable and implementation action plan are provided in Table 1.

DEFINING SERVICES AND METHODS

In most instances, but not all, the type of service to be offered has been identified before the initial staff meeting. If not, this should be completed within a week of the initial meeting. Sufficient market assessment data should be available at the first meeting so that discussion can begin and a decision can be reached at that time. The challenge lies in defining each service as a tangible product that can be described to and experienced by the patient. Whether the service is diabetes education, a weight-loss clinic, or a smoking cessation program, it must be spelled out in terms that the patient can understand. Remember that expressions such as "improved drug therapy outcomes" and "pharmaceutical care" are meaningless to patients.

Once the service has been defined, preparation for providing the service can actually begin. What methods will be employed to deliver the service? Will patient consultations occur on demand or by appointment? Will the pharmacist and patient stand or sit during the consultation? What will the pharmacist actually do when consulting with the patient? Answering these questions will help create a mental image of the service and determine the physical environment and resources needed to provide it.

Brochures, patient handouts, and educational media will need to be assembled to support the service. Files of information should be created, and methods established for acquiring and updating materials so they are readily accessible and can be easily shared with patients and stakeholders.

TABLE 1. SAMPLE IMPLEMENTATION ACTION PLAN AND TIMETABLE

Month	1				2				3				4				5				6			
Week	1	2	3	4	1	2	3	4	1	2	3	4	1	2	3	4	1	2	3	4	1	2	3	4
1.0 Establish goals	█																							
2.0 Define services and methods																								
2.1 Assess market	█																							
2.2 Develop care process	█	█																						
2.3 Assemble care resources	█	█																						
3.0 Workflow and staffing																								
3.1 Assess current processes			█																					
3.2 Estimate staffing needs			█																					
3.3 Recruit staff				█	█	█																		
3.4 Select transition day						█																		
4.0 Staff training																								
4.1 Determine needs					█																			
4.2 Select/outline methods					█																			
4.3 Conduct training					█	█	█	█	█	█	█	█	█											
5.0 Facility redesign																								
5.1 Draft plans			█																					
5.2 Hire contractor					█																			
5.3 Procure fixtures and equipment					█																			
5.4 Monitor construction						█	█	█	█	█	█	█	█											
6.0 Marketing																								
6.1 Develop plan					█																			
6.2 Carry out plan					█	█	█	█	█	█	█	█	█	█	█	█	█	█	█	█	█	█	█	█
7.0 Business plan																								
7.1 Estimate expenses/revenue					█																			
7.2 Track expenses/revenue						█	█	█	█	█	█	█	█	█	█	█	█	█	█	█	█	█	█	█

WORKFLOW AND STAFFING

Since the lack of time for patient interaction is the most frequently cited barrier to providing pharmaceutical care, staffing time must be analyzed thoroughly, as described in Chapter 7. During the first staff meeting, procedures that need to be followed and the rationale for each should be outlined. Everyone must cooperate and offer input so that current contributions of staff members can be estimated accurately—and also so that each person develops a sense of ownership toward the new practice.

After determining the pharmacy workflow (see page 120) and completing the Staffing Adjustment Worksheet (see page 123), it will likely be evident that changes in staffing and staff hours are necessary. New roles will probably need to be defined and responsibilities reassigned for various tasks related to dispensing and pharmacy operations.

TRANSITION DAY

A key step is choosing a "transition day" that marks the last day of the dispensing-oriented practice and the first day of the pharmaceutical care practice. (Think of it as similar to the "stop date" in a smoking cessation program.) The date should be as soon as possible—ideally, within a month of making the decision to change. This way, the staff's level of enthusiasm does not have time to drop. Some pharmacists may wish to wait until the facility redesign is completed, but this is not recommended. Ideas about the redesign may change as new staffing arrangements and workflow patterns get under way.

The transition day should be one that traditionally is less busy than others. Before that day, everyone on staff should be made aware that getting used to the new workflow will be a gradual process that can take as long as four months. The staff will need to experiment with different workflow patterns to find the one that works best. All staff must have a voice in the transition process and a stake in the pharmacy's success.

In the first days of the new practice, many pharmacists get an urge to return to the old workflow because they do not feel "busy" enough. This is a mistake, as cited by many pharmacists who reverted to their old ways. Keep in mind that implementing the new practice is a process, not a one-time event. Focus on goals for the future to avoid slipping back into familiar, comfortable work patterns.

Develop the habit of interacting with patients on the pharmacy floor. In the first weeks, focus on simple interactions, such as updating patient profiles, counseling about medications, and introducing the concept of pharmaceutical care. Pharmacists and patients must get used to interacting in a different location, and for a different purpose, than they did before.

STAFF TRAINING

The training needs of personnel should be addressed as soon as possible. Pharmacists will most likely need to learn about the pharmaceutical care process and will require opportunities to practice new patient care skills. Training courses in management skills may be helpful for both pharmacists and other supervisors. Technicians and clerks need to be taught dispensing tasks that have been newly delegated to them. So that scheduling is as flexible as possible, all staff should know how to read and process prescriptions.

Technicians should also learn to facilitate pharmacists' activities, such as printing out warning notices to be included with processed prescriptions that the pharmacist will eventually check. Protocols will need to be developed and put into use for responding appropriately to telephone prescription requests and addressing drug interaction warnings generated by the pharmacy's dispensing computer software. Technicians should also receive training in methods for resolving reimbursement problems.

When planning retraining, a choice must be made between on-the-job training or formal training programs. The training skills and knowledge of existing personnel must be factored into this decision. If existing staff possess the necessary skills to train other personnel, then in-house training may be a viable option. However, there must be adequate time for this training to occur. If enough time for training is not available during regular pharmacy hours, training may have to take place either before or after the normal work day. Staff may need to put in extra hours—which may mean providing them with extra pay.

If in-house training is decided on, procedures must be in place to assure that staff members can perform the new tasks proficiently. Options for testing the skills and knowledge of technicians include monitoring telephone communications, tracking dispensing accuracy, and observing patient interactions. The evaluation process should be ongoing and should provide constructive feedback to the staff to help them improve over time. If in-house training is not possible, the pharmacy may wish to take advantage of training resources at a local college.

Eventually it would be a good idea to have each technician seek certification to validate specific knowledge and skills. Certification is also beneficial for enhancing technicians' self-esteem and creating a more professional image for the pharmacy. Most state and national pharmacy associations can provide information about obtaining pharmacy technician certification.

FACILITY REDESIGN

After staff considerations have been addressed, the focus should be on procuring materials or fixtures for redesigning the facility. Local office

BASIC COMPONENTS OF A BUSINESS PLAN

Following are some key elements of a business plan. Keep in mind that this is not a comprehensive list. When developing a business plan, referring to business development texts readily available at libraries and bookstores may be worthwhile. Seeking assistance from experts in business development, accounting, and marketing may be useful, as well.

1. Executive summary highlighting major aspects of the plan

2. Description of the proposed services, including:
   - Scope of service
   - Benefits of the services and needs that will be met
   - Types of people to be served

3. Market analysis, including:
   - A profile of the target customer population
   - Potential sources of referrals
   - Market size and projected growth rates
   - Discussion of price-sensitivity issues

4. Marketing plan, including:
   - Target groups and tactics for promoting the service to them
   - Promotion schedule and approaches, such as open house, brochure mailing, physician office visits
   - Method for tracking results of promotions

5. Analysis of issues related to the facility and equipment, including:
   - Plans for renovation or redesign
   - Equipment requirements
   - Contingency plan for cost overruns
   - Regulatory requirements that must be met

6. Management and organization, including:
   - Organizational structure
   - Management capabilities and expertise needed
   - Staffing plan
   - Contractual relationships to put in place, if any
   - Implementation plan

7. Financial analysis, including:
   - Three- to five-year financial projections
   - Payer mix projected
   - Inflation factors
   - Costs of salaries and benefits
   - Nonwage costs
   - Break-even analysis
   - Capital costs, such as construction and equipment

8. Legal assessment, including:
   - Regulatory requirements
   - Licensure requirements
   - Contract review

9. Plan for evaluating the service after launch
   - Performance indicators, including financial, clinical, customer satisfaction
   - Time frame for evaluations

Source: Adapted from Flagstad MS. Identifying Profitable Areas of Expansion: Business Planning. Presented at the ASHP Second Annual Leadership Conference on Pharmacy Practice Management, Reston, VA, October 1997.

supply stores may stock inexpensive partitions and additional equipment or supplies, such as file cabinets and folders. Secondhand stores may offer inexpensive alternatives to new equipment. If renovations are planned, a contractor should be hired as soon as possible because delays are almost guaranteed. Be prepared to monitor the reconstruction process carefully.

MARKETING AND BUSINESS PLANS

Detailed marketing plans (see Chapter 9) and business plans are very important. The basic components of a good business plan are listed in the box on page 219. Pharmacists should definitely seek financial advice to help them estimate and track expenses and project revenues related to the new service. Understanding what is required financially to launch the pharmaceutical care practice and knowing when a return on investment can be realized will help avoid unrealistic financial expectations and promote sound business decisions.

STAYING ON TRACK

When implementing pharmaceutical care, the pharmacist should set reasonable goals with a reasonable time line and specific measurable endpoints. Weekly progress checks can ensure that the process is moving along. If goals are being met sooner than expected, or more slowly than desired, the schedule may need to be adjusted accordingly.

Supportive resources to help the pharmacist through the transition process are useful for keeping the plan on track. For example, pharmacists can seek advice from others who have already converted their practices and can obtain guidance from state professional associations or colleges of pharmacy. Another option is forming a "work group" of fellow pharmacists to serve as a forum for trouble-shooting and problem-solving. Communication venues such as Internet news groups, bulletin boards, and chat rooms are another option that can be explored for ongoing assistance and support.

CONCLUSION

The implementation process is simply that—a process. Successful implementation will take time, energy, and the redirection of goals and resources. Pharmacists, staff, patients, and prescribers will need to become acclimated to a new paradigm. With the right attitude, good planning, and adequate support, the goal of restructuring the pharmacy to provide pharmaceutical care will lead to a successful and rewarding practice.

REFERENCE

1. Covey SR. *The Seven Habits of Highly Effective People*. New York: Simon and Schuster; 1989.

Appendix A

♦

Principles of Practice for Pharmaceutical Care

♦

American Pharmaceutical Association

PREAMBLE

Pharmaceutical care is a patient-centered, outcomes oriented pharmacy practice that requires the pharmacist to work in concert with the patient and the patient's other healthcare providers to promote health, to prevent disease, and to assess, monitor, initiate, and modify medication use to assure that drug therapy[1] regimens are safe and effective. The goal of pharmaceutical care is to optimize the patient's health-related quality of life, and achieve positive clinical outcomes, within realistic economic expenditures. To achieve this goal, the following must be accomplished:

A. A PROFESSIONAL RELATIONSHIP MUST BE ESTABLISHED AND MAINTAINED.

Interaction between the pharmacist and the patient must occur to assure that a relationship based upon caring, trust, open communication, cooperation, and mutual decision making is established and maintained. In this relationship, the pharmacist holds the patient's welfare paramount, maintains an appropriate attitude of caring for the patient's welfare, and uses all his/her professional knowledge and skills on the patient's behalf. In exchange, the patient agrees to supply personal information and preferences, and participate in the therapeutic plan. The pharmacist develops mechanisms to assure the patient has access to pharmaceutical care at all times.

B. PATIENT-SPECIFIC MEDICAL INFORMATION MUST BE COLLECTED, ORGANIZED, RECORDED, AND MAINTAINED.

Pharmacists must collect and/or generate subjective and objective information regarding the patient's general health and activity status, past medical history, medication history, social history, diet and exercise history, history of present illness, and economic situation (financial and insured status). Sources of information may include, but are not limited to, the patient, medical charts and reports, pharmacist-conducted health/physical assessment, the patient's family or caregiver, insurer, and other healthcare providers

---

1. Although "drug therapy" typically refers to intended, beneficial effects of pharmacologic drugs, in this document, "drug therapy" refers to the intended, beneficial use of drugs—whether diagnostic or therapeutic—and thus includes diagnostic radiopharmaceuticals, X-ray contrast media, etc. in addition to pharmacologic drugs. Similarly, "drug therapy plan" includes the outcomes-oriented plan for diagnostic drug use in addition to pharmacologic drug use.

including physicians, nurses, mid level practitioners and other pharmacists. Since this information will form the basis for decisions regarding the development and subsequent modification of the drug therapy plan, it must be timely, accurate, and complete, and it must be organized and recorded to assure that it is readily retrievable and updated as necessary and appropriate. Patient information must be maintained in a confidential manner.

C. PATIENT-SPECIFIC MEDICAL INFORMATION MUST BE EVALUATED AND A DRUG THERAPY PLAN DEVELOPED MUTUALLY WITH THE PATIENT.

Based upon a thorough understanding of the patient and his/her condition or disease and its treatment, the pharmacist must, with the patient and with the patient's other healthcare providers as necessary, develop an outcomes-oriented drug therapy plan. The plan may have various components which address each of the patient's diseases or conditions. In designing the plan, the pharmacist must carefully consider the psychosocial aspects of the disease as well as the potential relationship between the cost and/or complexity of therapy and patient adherence. As one of the patient's advocates, the pharmacist assures the coordination of drug therapy with the patient's other healthcare providers and the patient. In addition, the patient must be apprised of (1) various pros and cons (i.e., cost, side effects, different monitoring aspects, etc.) of the options relative to drug therapy and (2) instances where one option may be more beneficial based on the pharmacist's professional judgment. The essential elements of the plan, including the patient's responsibilities, must be carefully and completely explained to the patient. Information should be provided to the patient at a level the patient will understand. The drug therapy plan must be documented in the patient's pharmacy record and communicated to the patient's other healthcare providers as necessary.

D. THE PHARMACIST ASSURES THAT THE PATIENT HAS ALL SUPPLIES, INFORMATION, AND KNOWLEDGE NECESSARY TO CARRY OUT THE DRUG THERAPY PLAN.

The pharmacist providing pharmaceutical care must assume ultimate responsibility for assuring that his/her patient has been able to obtain, and is appropriately using, any drugs and related products or equipment called for in the drug therapy plan. The pharmacist must also assure that the patient has a thorough understanding of the disease and the therapy/medications prescribed in the plan.

E. THE PHARMACIST REVIEWS, MONITORS, AND MODIFIES THE THERAPEUTIC PLAN AS NECESSARY AND APPROPRIATE, IN CONCERT WITH THE PATIENT AND HEALTHCARE TEAM.

The pharmacist is responsible for monitoring the patient's progress in achieving the specific outcomes according to strategy developed in the drug therapy plan. The pharmacist coordinates changes in the plan with the patient and the patient's other healthcare providers as necessary and appropriate in order to maintain or enhance the safety and/or effectiveness of drug therapy and to help minimize overall healthcare costs. Patient progress is accurately documented in the pharmacy record and communicated to the patient and to the patient's other healthcare providers as appropriate. The pharmacist shares information with other healthcare providers as the setting for care changes, thus helping assure continuity of care as the patient moves between the community setting, the institutional setting, and the long-term care setting.

PRACTICE PRINCIPLES

1. DATA COLLECTION

1.1 The pharmacist conducts an initial interview with the patient for the purposes of establishing a professional working relationship and initiating the patient's pharmacy record. In some situations (e.g., pediatrics, geriatrics, critical care, language barriers) the opportunity to develop a professional relationship with and collect information directly from the patient may not exist. Under these circumstances, the pharmacist should work directly with the patient's parent, guardian, and/or principal caregiver.

1.2 The interview is organized, professional, and meets the patient's need for confidentiality and privacy. Adequate time is devoted to assure that questions and answers can be fully developed without either party feeling uncomfortable or hurried. The interview is used to systematically collect patient-specific subjective information and to initiate a pharmacy record which includes information and data regarding the patient's general health and activity status, past medical history, medication history, social history (including economic situation), family history, and history of present illness. The record should also include information regarding the patient's thoughts or feelings and perceptions of his/her condition or disease.

1.3 The pharmacist uses health/physical assessment techniques (blood-pressure monitoring, etc.) appropriately and as necessary to acquire necessary patient-specific objective information.

1.4 The pharmacist uses appropriate secondary sources to supplement the information obtained through the initial patient interview and health/physical assessment. Sources may include, but are not limited to, the patient's medical record or medical reports, the patient's family, and the patient's other healthcare providers.

1.5 The pharmacist creates a pharmacy record for the patient and accurately records the information collected. The pharmacist assures that the patient's record is appropriately organized, kept current, and accurately reflects all pharmacist-patient encounters. The confidentiality of the information in the record is carefully guarded and appropriate systems are in place to assure security. Patient-identifiable information contained in the record is provided to others only upon the authorization of the patient or as required by law.

2. INFORMATION EVALUATION

2.1 The pharmacist evaluates the subjective and objective information collected from the patient and other sources then forms conclusions regarding: (1) opportunities to improve and/or assure the safety, effectiveness, and/or economy of current or planned drug therapy; (2) opportunities to minimize current or potential future drug or health-related problems; and (3) the timing of any necessary future pharmacist consultation.

2.2 The pharmacist records the conclusions of the evaluation in the medical and/or pharmacy record.

2.3 The pharmacist discusses the conclusions with the patient, as necessary and appropriate, and assures an appropriate understanding of the nature of the condition or illness and what might be expected with respect to its management.

3. FORMULATING A PLAN

3.1 The pharmacist, in concert with other healthcare providers, identifies, evaluates, and then chooses the most appropriate action(s) to: (1) improve and/or assure the safety, effectiveness, and/or cost-effectiveness of current or planned drug therapy; and/or (2) minimize current or potential future health-related problems.

3.2 The pharmacist formulates plans to effect the desired outcome. The plans may include, but are not limited to, work with the patient as well as with other health providers to develop a patient-specific drug therapy protocol or to modify prescribed drug therapy, develop and/or implement drug therapy monitoring mechanisms, recommend nutritional or dietary modifications, add nonprescription medications or nondrug treatments, refer the patient to an appropriate source of care, or institute an existing drug therapy protocol.

3.3 For each problem identified, the pharmacist actively considers the patient's needs and determines the desirable and mutually agreed upon outcome and incorporates these into the plan. The plan may include specific disease state and drug therapy endpoints and monitoring endpoints.

3.4 The pharmacist reviews the plan and desirable outcomes with the patient and with the patient's other healthcare provider(s) as appropriate.

3.5 The pharmacist documents the plan and desirable outcomes in the patient's medical and/or pharmacy record.

4. Implementing the Plan

4.1 The pharmacist and the patient take the steps necessary to implement the plan. These steps may include, but are not limited to, contacting other health providers to clarify or modify prescriptions, initiating drug therapy, educating the patient and/or caregiver(s), coordinating the acquisition of medications and/or related supplies, which might include helping the patient overcome financial barriers or lifestyle barriers that might otherwise interfere with the therapy plan, or coordinating appointments with other healthcare providers to whom the patient is being referred.

4.2 The pharmacist works with the patient to maximize patient understanding and involvement in the therapy plan, assures that arrangements for drug therapy monitoring (e.g., laboratory evaluation, blood pressure monitoring, home blood glucose testing, etc.) are made and understood by the patient, and that the patient receives and knows how to properly use all necessary medications and related equipment. Explanations are tailored to the patient's level of comprehension and teaching and adherence aids are employed as indicated.

4.3 The pharmacist assures that appropriate mechanisms are in place to ensure that the proper medications, equipment, and supplies are received by the patient in a timely fashion.

4.4 The pharmacist documents in the medical and/or pharmacy record the steps taken to implement the plan including the appropriate baseline monitoring parameters, and any barriers which will need to be overcome.

4.5 The pharmacist communicates the elements of the plan to the patient and/or the patient's other healthcare provider(s). The pharmacist shares information with other healthcare providers as the setting for care changes, in order to help maintain continuity of care as the patient moves between the ambulatory, inpatient, or long-term care environment.

5. Monitoring and Modifying the Plan/Assuring Positive Outcomes

5.1 The pharmacist regularly reviews subjective and objective monitoring parameters in order to determine if satisfactory progress is being made toward achieving desired outcomes as outlined in the drug therapy plan.

5.2 The pharmacist and patient determine if the original plan should continue to be followed or if modifications are needed. If changes are necessary, the pharmacist works with the patient/caregiver and his/her other healthcare providers to modify and implement the revised plan as described in "Formulating a Plan" and "Implementing the Plan" above.

5.3 The pharmacist reviews ongoing progress in achieving desired outcomes with the patient and provides a report to the patient's other healthcare providers as appropriate. As progress towards outcomes is achieved, the pharmacist should provide positive reinforcement.

5.4 A mechanism is established for follow-up with patients. The pharmacist uses appropriate professional judgment in determining the need to notify the patient's other healthcare providers of the patient's level of adherence with the plan.

5.5 The pharmacist updates the patient's medical and/or pharmacy record with information concerning patient progress, noting the subjective and objective information which has been considered, his/her assessment of the patient's current progress, the patient's assessment of his/her current progress, and any modifications that are being made to the plan. Communications with other healthcare providers should also be noted.

Appendix

Pharmaceutical care is a process of drug therapy management that requires a change in the orientation of traditional professional attitudes and re-engineering of the traditional pharmacy environment. Certain elements of structure must be in place to provide quality pharmaceutical care. Some of these elements are: (1) knowledge, skill, and function of personnel, (2) systems for data collection, documentation, and transfer of information, (3) efficient work flow processes, (4) references, resources, and equipment, (5) communication skills, and (6) commitment to quality improvement and assessment procedures.

Knowledge, skill, and function of personnel

The implementation of pharmaceutical care is supported by knowledge and skills in the area of patient assessment, clinical information, communication, adult teaching and learning principles, and psychosocial aspects of care. To use these skills, responsibilities must be reassessed, and assigned to appropriate personnel, including pharmacists, technicians, automation, and technology. A mechanism of certifying and credentialling will support the implementation of pharmaceutical care.

Systems for data collection and documentation

The implementation of pharmaceutical care is supported by data collection and documentation systems that accommodate patient care communications (e.g., patient contact notes, medical/medication history), interprofessional communications (e.g., physician communication, pharmacist to pharmacist communication), quality assurance (e.g., patient outcomes assessment, patient care protocols), and research (e.g., data for pharmacoepidemiology, etc.). Documentation systems are vital for reimbursement considerations.

Efficient work flow processes

The implementation of pharmaceutical care is supported by incorporating patient care into the activities of the pharmacist and other personnel.

References, resources, and equipment

The implementation of pharmaceutical care is supported by tools which facilitate patient care, including equipment to assess medication therapy adherence and effectiveness, clinical resource materials, and patient education materials. Tools may include computer software support, drug utilization evaluation (DUE) programs, disease management protocols, etc.

Communication skills

The implementation of pharmaceutical care is supported by patient-centered communication. Within this communication, the patient plays a key role in the overall management of the therapy plan.

Quality assessment/improvement programs

The implementation and practice of pharmaceutical care is supported and improved by measuring, assessing, and improving pharmaceutical care activities utilizing the conceptual framework of continuous quality improvement.

NOTE: This document will not cover each and every situation; that was not the intent of the Advisory Committee. This is a dynamic document and is intended to be revised as the profession adapts to its new role. It is hoped that pharmacists will use these principles, adapting them to their own situation and environments, to establish and implement pharmaceutical care.

Prepared by the APhA Pharmaceutical Care Guidelines Advisory Committee; approved by the APhA Board of Trustees, August 1995. © 1996 by the American Pharmaceutical Association. All rights reserved.

Appendix B

◆

American Society of Health-System Pharmacists Statement on Pharmaceutical Care

The purpose of this statement is to assist pharmacists in understanding pharmaceutical care. Such understanding must precede efforts to implement pharmaceutical care, which ASHP believes merit the highest priority in all practice settings.

Possibly the earliest published use of the term pharmaceutical care was by Brodie in the context of thoughts about drug use control and medication-related services.[1,2] It is a term that has been widely used and a concept about which much has been written and discussed in the pharmacy profession, especially since the publication of a paper by Hepler and Strand in 1990.[3-5] ASHP has formally endorsed the concept.[6] With varying terminology and nuances, the concept has also been acknowledged by other national pharmacy organizations.[7,8] Implementation of pharmaceutical care was the focus of a major ASHP conference in March 1993.

Many pharmacists have expressed enthusiasm for the concept of pharmaceutical care, but there has been substantial inconsistency in its description. Some have characterized it as merely a new name for clinical pharmacy; others have described it as anything that pharmacists do that may lead to beneficial results for patients.

ASHP believes that pharmaceutical care is an important new concept that represents growth in the profession beyond clinical pharmacy as often practiced and beyond other activities of pharmacists, including medication preparation and dispensing. All of these professional activities are important, however, and ASHP continues to be a strong proponent of the necessity for pharmacists' involvement in them. In practice, these activities should be integrated with and culminate in pharmaceutical care provided by individual pharmacists to individual patients.

In 1992, ASHP's members urged the development of an officially recognized ASHP definition of pharmaceutical care.[9] This statement provides a definition and elucidates some of the elements and implications of that definition. The definition that follows is an adaptation of a definition developed by Hepler and Strand.[3]

DEFINITION

The mission of the pharmacist is to provide pharmaceutical care. Pharmaceutical care is the direct, responsible provision of medication-related care for the purpose of achieving definite outcomes that improve a patient's quality of life.

PRINCIPAL ELEMENTS

The principal elements of pharmaceutical care are that it is *medication related*; it is *care* that is *directly provided* to the patient; it is provided to produce *definite outcomes*; these outcomes are intended to improve the patient's *quality of life*; and the provider accepts personal *responsibility* for the outcomes.

Medication Related. Pharmaceutical care involves not only medication therapy (the actual provision of medication) but also decisions about medication use for individual patients. As appropriate, this includes decisions *not* to use medication therapy as well as judgments about medication selection, dosages, routes and methods of administration, medication therapy monitoring, and the provision of medication-related information and counseling to individual patients.

Care. Central to the concept of care is caring, a personal concern for the well-being of another person. Overall patient care consists of integrated domains of care including (among others) medical care, nursing care, and pharmaceutical care. Health professionals in each of these disciplines possess unique expertise and must cooperate in the patient's overall care. At times, they share in the execution of the various types of care (including pharmaceutical care). To pharmaceutical care, however, the pharmacist contributes unique knowledge and skills to ensure optimal outcomes from the use of medications.

At the heart of any type of patient care, there exists a one-to-one relationship between a caregiver and a patient. In pharmaceutical care, the irreducible "unit" of care is one pharmacist in a direct professional relationship with one patient. In this relationship, the pharmacist provides care directly to the patient and for the benefit of the patient.

The health and well-being of the patient are paramount. The pharmacist makes a direct, personal, caring commitment to the individual patient and acts in the patient's best interest. The pharmacist cooperates directly with other professionals and the patient in designing, implementing, and monitoring a therapeutic plan intended to produce definite therapeutic outcomes that improve the patient's quality of life.

Outcomes. It is the goal of pharmaceutical care to improve an individual patient's quality of life through achievement of definite (predefined), medication-related therapeutic outcomes. The outcomes sought are:

1. Cure of a patient's disease.

2. Elimination or reduction of a patient's symptomatology.

3. Arresting or slowing of a disease process.

4. Preventing a disease or symptomatology.

This, in turn, involves three major functions: (1) identifying potential and actual medication-related problems, (2) resolving actual medication-related problems, and (3) preventing potential medication-related problems. A medication-related problem is an event or circumstance involving medication therapy that actually or potentially interferes with an optimum outcome for a specific patient. There are at least the following categories of medication-related problems:[3]

- *Untreated indications.* The patient has a medical problem that requires medication therapy (an indication for medication use) but is not receiving a medication for that indication.

- *Improper drug selection.* The patient has a medication indication but is taking the wrong medication.

- *Subtherapeutic dosage.* The patient has a medical problem that is being treated with too little of the correct medication.

- **Failure to receive medication.** The patient has a medical problem that is the result of not receiving a medication (e.g., for pharmaceutical, psychological, sociological, or economic reasons).

- **Overdosage.** The patient has a medical problem that is being treated with too much of the correct medication (toxicity).

- **Adverse drug reactions.** The patient has a medical problem that is the result of an adverse drug reaction or adverse effect.

- **Drug interactions.** The patient has a medical problem that is the result of a drug-drug, drug-food, or drug-laboratory test interaction.

- **Medication use without indication.** The patient is taking a medication for no medically valid indication.

Patients may possess characteristics that interfere with the achievement of desired therapeutic outcomes. Patients may be noncompliant with prescribed medication use regimens, or there may be unpredictable variation in patients' biological responses. Thus, in an imperfect world, intended outcomes from medication-related therapy are not always achievable.

Patients bear a responsibility to help achieve the desired outcomes by engaging in behaviors that will contribute to—and not interfere with—the achievement of desired outcomes. Pharmacists and other health professionals have an obligation to educate patients about behaviors that will contribute to achieving desired outcomes.

Quality of Life. Some tools exist now for assessing a patient's quality of life. These tools are still evolving, and pharmacists should maintain familiarity with the literature on this subject.[10,11] A complete assessment of a patient's quality of life should include both objective and subjective (e.g., the patient's own) assessments. Patients should be involved, in an informed way, in establishing quality-of-life goals for their therapies.

Responsibility. The fundamental relationship in any type of patient care is a mutually beneficial exchange in which the patient grants authority to the provider and the provider gives competence and commitment to the patient (accepts responsibility).[3] Responsibility involves both moral trustworthiness and accountability.

In pharmaceutical care, the direct relationship between an individual pharmacist and an individual patient is that of a professional covenant in which the patient's safety and well-being are entrusted to the pharmacist, who commits to honoring that trust through competent professional actions that are in the patient's best interest. As an accountable member of the health-care team, the pharmacist must document the care provided.[4,7,12,13] The pharmacist is personally accountable for patient outcomes (the quality of care) that ensue from the pharmacist's actions and decisions.[1]

IMPLICATIONS

The idea that pharmacists should commit themselves to the achievement of definite outcomes for individual patients is an especially important element in the concept of pharmaceutical care. The expectation that pharmacists personally accept responsibility for individual patients' outcomes that result from the pharmacists' actions represents a significant advance in pharmacy's continuing professionalization. The provision of pharmaceutical care represents a maturation of pharmacy as a clinical profession and is a natural evolution of more mature clinical pharmacy activities of pharmacists.[14]

ASHP believes that pharmaceutical care is fundamental to the profession's purpose of helping people make the best use of medications.[15] It is a unifying concept that transcends all types of patients and all categories of pharmacists and pharmacy organizations. Pharmaceutical care is applicable and achievable by pharmacists in all practice settings. The provision of pharmaceutical care is not limited to pharmacists in inpatient, outpatient, or community settings, nor to pharmacists with certain degrees, specialty certifications, residencies, or other credentials. It is not limited to those in academic or teaching settings. Pharmaceutical care is not a matter of formal credentials or place of work. Rather, it is a matter of a direct personal, professional, responsible relationship with a patient to ensure that the patient's use of medication is optimal and leads to improvements in the patient's quality of life.

Pharmacists should commit themselves to continuous care on behalf of individual patients. They bear responsibility for ensuring that the patient's care is ongoing despite work-shift changes, weekends, and holidays. An important implication is that a pharmacist providing pharmaceutical care may need to work as a member of a team of pharmacists who provide backup care when the primary responsible pharmacist is not available. Another is that the responsible pharmacist should work to ensure that continuity of care is maintained when a patient moves from one component of a health-care system to another (e.g., when a patient is hospitalized or discharged from a hospital to return to an ambulatory, community status). In the provision of pharmaceutical care, professional communication about the patient's needs between responsible pharmacists in each area of practice is, therefore, essential. ASHP believes that the development of recognized methods of practicing pharmaceutical care that will enhance such communication is an important priority for the profession.

Pharmaceutical care can be conceived as both a purpose for pharmacy practice and a purpose of medication use processes. That is, a fundamental professional reason that pharmacists engage in pharmacy practice should be to deliver pharmaceutical care. Furthermore, the medication use systems that pharmacists (and others) operate should be designed to support and enable the delivery of pharmaceutical care by individual pharmacists. ASHP believes that, in organized health-care settings, pharmaceutical care can be most successfully provided when it is part of the pharmacy department's central mission and when management activity is focused on facilitating the provision of pharmaceutical care by individual pharmacists. This approach, in which empowered frontline staff provide direct care to individual patients and are supported by managers, other pharmacists, and support systems, is new for many pharmacists and managers.

An important corollary to this approach is that pharmacists providing pharmaceutical care in organized health-care settings cannot provide such care alone. They must work in an interdependent fashion with colleagues in pharmacy and other disciplines, support systems and staff, and managers.[7] It is incumbent upon pharmacists to design work systems and practices that appropriately focus the efforts of all activities and support systems on meeting the needs of patients. Some patients will require different levels of care, and it may be useful to structure work systems in light of those differences.[16,17] ASHP believes that the provision of pharmaceutical care and the development of effective work systems to document and support it are major priorities for the profession.

In the provision of pharmaceutical care, pharmacists use their unique perspective and knowledge of medication therapy to evaluate patients' actual and potential medication-related problems. To do this, they require direct access to clinical information about individual patients. They make judgments regarding medication use and then advocate optimal medication use for individual patients in cooperation with other professionals and in consideration of their unique professional knowledge and evaluations. Pharmaceutical care includes the active participation of the patient (and designated caregivers such as family members) in matters pertinent to medication use.

The acknowledgment of pharmacists' responsibility for therapeutic outcomes resulting from their actions does not contend that pharmacists have exclusive authority for matters related to medication use. Other health-care professionals, including physicians and nurses, have valuable and well-established, well-recognized roles in the medication use process. The pharmaceutical care concept does not diminish the roles or responsibilities of other health professionals, nor does it imply any usurping of authority by pharmacists. Pharmacists' actions in pharmaceutical care should be conducted and viewed as collaborative. The knowledge, skills, and traditions of pharmacists, however, make them legitimate leaders of efforts by health-care teams to improve patients' medication use.

Pharmaceutical care requires a direct relationship between a pharmacist and an individual patient. Some pharmacists and other pharmacy personnel engage in clinical and product-related pharmacy activities that do not involve a direct relationship with the patient. Properly designed, these activities can be supportive of pharmaceutical care, but ASHP believes it would be confusing and counterproductive to characterize such activities as pharmaceutical care. ASHP believes that clinical and product-related pharmacy activities are essential, however, and are as important as the actions of pharmacists interacting directly with patients.

Pharmaceutical educators must teach pharmaceutical care to students.[18] Providers of continuing education should help practicing pharmacists and other pharmacy personnel understand pharmaceutical care. Students and pharmacists should be taught to conceptualize and execute responsible medication-related problem-solving on behalf of individual patients. Curricula should be designed to produce graduates with sufficient knowledge and skills to provide pharmaceutical care competently.[8,18] Initiatives are under way to bring about these changes.[8] Practicing pharmacists must commit their time as preceptors and their workplaces as teaching laboratories for the undergraduate and postgraduate education and training necessary to produce pharmacists who can provide pharmaceutical care.[8]

Research is needed to evaluate various methods and systems for the delivery of pharmaceutical care.

Pharmaceutical care represents an exciting new vision for pharmacy. ASHP hopes that all pharmacists in all practice settings share in this vision and that the pharmaceutical care concept will serve as a stimulus for them to work toward transforming the profession to actualize that vision.

REFERENCES

1. Brodie DC. Is pharmaceutical education prepared to lead its profession? The Ninth Annual Rho Chi Lecture. *Rep Rho Chi.* 1973;39:6-12.

2. Brodie DC, Parish PA, Poston JW. Societal needs for drugs and drug-related services. *Am J Pharm Educ.* 1980;44:276-8.

3. Hepler CD, Strand LM. Opportunities and responsibilities in pharmaceutical care. *Am J Hosp Pharm.* 1990;47:533-43.

4. Penna RP. Pharmaceutical care: pharmacy's mission for the 1990s. *Am J Hosp Pharm.* 1990;47:543-9.

5. Pierpaoli PG, Hethcox JM. Pharmaceutical care: new management and leadership imperatives. *Top Hosp Pharm Manage.* 1992;12:1-18.

6. Oddis JA. Report of the House of Delegates: June 3 and 5, 1991. *Am J Hosp Pharm.* 1991;48:1739-48.

7. American Pharmaceutical Association. An APhA white paper on the role of the pharmacist in comprehensive medication use management; the delivery of pharmaceutical care. Washington, DC: American Pharmaceutical Association; March 1992.

8. Commission to Implement Change in Pharmaceutical Education. A position paper. Entry-level education in pharmacy: a commitment to change. *AACP News.* 1991;Nov (Suppl):14.

9. Oddis JA. Report of the House of Delegates: June 1 and 3, 1992. *Am J Hosp Pharm.* 1992;49:1962-73.

10. Gouveia WA. Measuring and managing patient outcomes. *Am J Hosp Pharm.* 1992; 49:2157-8.

11. MacKeigan LD, Pathak DS. Overview of health-related quality-of-life measures. *Am J Hosp Pharm.* 1992;49:2236-45.

12. Galinsky RE, Nickman NA. Pharmacists and the mandate of pharmaceutical care. *DICP Ann Pharmacother.* 1991;21:431-4.

13. Angaran DM. Quality assurance to quality improvement: measuring and monitoring pharmaceutical care. *Am J Hosp Pharm.* 1991;48:1901-7.

14. Hepler CD. Pharmaceutical care and specialty practice. *Pharmacotherapy.* 1993; 13:64S-9S.

15. Zellmer WA. Expressing the mission of pharmacy practice. *Am J Hosp Pharm.* 1991; 48:1195. Editorial.

16. Smith WE, Benderev K. Levels of pharmaceutical care: a theoretical model. *Am J Hosp Pharm.*1991;48:540-6.

17. Strand LM, Cipolle RJ, Morley PC, et al. Levels of pharmaceutical care: a needs-based approach. *Am J Hosp Pharm.* 1991;48:547-50.

18. O'Neil EH. Health professions education for the future: schools in service to the nation. San Francisco, CA: Pew Health Profession Commission; 1993.

Index